Kicking Butts

Kicking Butts

Quit Smoking and
Take Charge of Your Health

SECOND EDITION

American Cancer Society®

Published by the American Cancer Society/Health Promotions
250 Williams Street NW
Atlanta, Georgia 30303-1002, USA

Printed in the United States of America
Composition by Graphic Composition, Inc.
Cover design by Elaine Callahan

5 4 3 2 1   10 11 12 13 14

Library of Congress Cataloging-in-Publication Data

Kicking butts : quit smoking and take charge of your health.—2nd ed.
       p. cm.
Includes bibliographical references and index.
ISBN-13: 978-1-60443-006-6 (pbk.: alk. paper)
ISBN-10: 1-60443-006-0 (pbk.: alk. paper)
1. Nicotine addiction—Treatment. 2. Smoking cessation. 3. Smoking—Health aspects. I. American Cancer Society.
   RA567.K53 2010
   613.85—dc22

                                                                        2010003703

AMERICAN CANCER SOCIETY
Managing Director, Content Chuck Westbrook
Director, Cancer Information Terri Ades, DNP, FNP-BC, AOCN
Director, Book Publishing Len Boswell
Managing Editor, Books Rebecca Teaff, MA
Books Editor Jill Russell
Book Publishing Coordinator Vanika Jordan, MSPub
Editorial Assistant, Books Amy Rovere

For more information, contact your American Cancer Society at **800-227-2345** or **cancer.org**.

Quantity discounts on bulk purchases of this book are available. Book excerpts can also be created to fit specific needs. For information, please contact the American Cancer Society, Health Promotions Publishing, 250 Williams Street NW, Atlanta, GA 30303-1002, or send an e-mail to **trade.sales@cancer.org**.

A Note to the Reader

The information contained in this book is not intended as medical advice and should not be relied upon as a substitute for talking with your doctor. All matters regarding your health require the supervision of a medical doctor who is familiar with your medical needs.

For more information, contact your American Cancer Society at **800-227-2345** (**cancer.org**).

Table of Contents

Introduction

YOU KNOW CIGARETTES AREN'T GOOD for you, but there's something about them that keeps you coming back. What is it that keeps you smoking? And what can help you stop?

This book will help you get to know your enemy, the cigarette, and learn what it takes to defeat it. After you are armed with this knowledge, you will experience one of the most important days in your life—the day you quit smoking.

You're Not Alone

Congratulations! Wanting to quit is an important first step. So now what? How do you quit and what should you do to keep from smoking again? Don't worry, we'll get to all of that, a little at a time.

Quitting smoking can be a real challenge, but you don't have to face it alone. We're going to be here every step of the way, pointing out hurdles to quitting and helping you over them. We'll show you lots of ways to help yourself quit.

By reading this book, you're taking control of the dangerous habit that has seeped into your life one puff at a time. Stick with us: We'll help you turn the tables and kick cigarette butts out of your life for good.

And it all begins here!

Know Your Enemy

The worst enemy is one that poses as a friend and fools you into becoming involved with it. This is just what cigarettes do. So why is something so harmful so hard to leave behind? Because powerful weapons keep you attached to cigarettes. Nicotine, peer pressure, habit, routine, and emotions all play a part in keeping you tied to smoking.

But you *can* quit. You're in control. As you understand more clearly why you smoke and how to break the cycle, you're more likely to kick the cigarette habit for good.

Anyone Can Kick the Tobacco Habit

Smokers aren't the only ones who want to kick tobacco out of their lives. People who chew tobacco, use snuff, or smoke cigars or pipes may also want to quit. Most tobacco users smoke cigarettes, so we focus on cigarette smoking in this book. But the information in *Kicking Butts* can help you no matter what type of tobacco you use. It can also help you help a friend or loved one quit using tobacco.

If You've Tried to Quit Before

You may be one of the many people who have tried to quit before. Having some past attempts under your belt can be a big help. Each time you try to quit, you learn what works and what doesn't work for you.

We'll help you look at past quit attempts and figure out what worked and what didn't. And we'll help get you ready to face situations like the one when you started smoking again—without smoking this time.

Your Plan of Attack

There is no one right way to quit smoking. People are different. They smoke for different reasons and have different reasons for wanting to stop. It may take some trial and error to find the combination of quitting options that's right for you. We'll outline all of your options. No matter which route you choose, all that matters is that it works for you.

Medications can help many people quit. Counseling and support from others help even more. You're most likely to quit for good if you use a combination of methods.

Each year, more than a million Americans stop smoking forever. You can be one of them. *Kicking Butts* will walk you through each step of quitting smoking.

How *Kicking Butts* Is Organized

In this book, we'll guide you through your quitting options, including medication and support. Then you can explore simple ways to cope with stress, face cravings, keep active, and stay determined. The information and worksheets will help guide you through your Quit Day . . . and your life as a nonsmoker.

Chapter 1: Facing the Challenges of Quitting

Knowing the challenges of how to stop smoking and getting ready for them will help as you quit. This chapter helps you learn why you smoke, the advantages of having tried to quit before, and how to overcome any doubts and fears about quitting. You'll be able to review your personal reasons for quitting, read about withdrawal symptoms, and make a commitment to quit.

Chapter 2: How to Quit: It's Up to You

Nicotine, an ingredient in tobacco products, can cause cravings in people who stop using tobacco. The withdrawal from nicotine pulls a lot of people back into smoking. You'll be glad to know that there are safe and effective ways to cut down on cravings and gradually break your body's reliance on nicotine. In this chapter, you'll learn about your many options for stop-smoking medications, which help many people kick the habit of smoking for good. You'll also learn about other methods of quitting and choices of support that can help.

Chapter 3: Countdown to Quitting

As you get ready to quit, you'll find suggestions for how to be with friends or loved ones who smoke; ideas for healthy eating, staying active, and coping with stress; and exactly what you can put in your "Bag of Tricks" (page 75) to get you through Quit Day and beyond as a proud nonsmoker.

Chapter 4: Quit Day

Chapter 4 outlines what to concentrate on during your Quit Day and will help you put your plans from previous chapters into motion. It also includes practical ideas for creating a smoke-free environment, facing cravings on Quit Day, and finding activities to keep your mind off smoking.

Chapter 5: Your Smoke-Free Life

Sometimes, reminders can keep you focused as you face each day as a nonsmoker. This chapter helps you look to the future, so you will be more prepared to face tempting situations without smoking. It will also cover how to learn from cravings. You're no doubt determined to make this quit attempt your last. But, if you do smoke after your Quit Day, Chapter 5 also addresses how to handle the setback.

A Helping Hand

This section is offered to those who would like to learn how to support a loved one who is trying to quit smoking. It is an easy-to-read list of tips for friends and loved ones to keep at hand.

Resource Guide

The American Cancer Society offers programs and services for people interested in quitting smoking. You can find overviews of the Society's and other organizations' important resources and contact information in the back of the book.

Glossary

A glossary of terms related to smoking cessation is included in the back of the book.

1

Facing the Challenges of Quitting

Q UITTING SMOKING ISN'T EASY. But together we are going to work through the challenges of quitting so you'll be prepared to make your quitting experience as simple as possible.

Most people start smoking when they're young and keep smoking because they like it. They may also like the way nicotine affects their bodies, even if they don't know exactly what it does. People may use nicotine to cope with stress, or they may smoke simply out of habit. In time, some smokers come to feel that smoking is part of every aspect of their lives. But the biggest reason most people continue to smoke—whether they realize it or not—is that they've become addicted to the nicotine in tobacco.

Some strong forces may be keeping *you* smoking— nicotine, the habit of smoking, a psychological or emotional attachment to smoking, or all of these things.

Yes, You *Can* Do It

Here's good news you can believe: *You can quit.* Remember, more than a million people do it every year. Anyone can do it, and if you plan for the bumps along the way, you can become a nonsmoker.

Nicotine Is a Drug

It may be hard to think of nicotine as a dangerous drug. Everybody knows nicotine products can be bought legally by adults at grocery stores, at corner stores, or even on the Internet. And you can't really see, smell, or taste the drug nicotine, which is found naturally in tobacco. But nicotine is a powerful drug with serious effects.

It's Addictive

The nicotine in cigarette smoke is what causes an addiction to smoking. Smoking isn't always something people continue to do by choice—even if they don't realize they're hooked on the drug. But, *like heroin and cocaine, nicotine is addictive.* To understand why, take a look at some facts about nicotine and how it tricks your body into thinking it needs it:

- When taken in small amounts, nicotine makes smokers feel good so they want to smoke more.

- Smokers usually become dependent on nicotine and feel withdrawal symptoms when they stop smoking. When people quit and feel bad, they're tempted to begin smoking again.

- Because nicotine affects the chemistry of the brain and central nervous system, smokers may rely on cigarettes to regulate their moods.

As with many addictive drugs, people develop a life-long dependence on nicotine. This means that when an ex-smoker smokes a cigarette, even years after quitting, it can trigger a nicotine reaction, hooking the person back into the habit of smoking again. At some point after you quit, you may get overconfident and think you can handle just one cigarette. Well, just one can be enough to send you right back to your old "pal" nicotine for another long-term visit. Since you don't want all your hard work to go to waste, we'll talk in Chapter 3 about exactly how to cope with everyday stresses without smoking.

People who have already quit smoking say that, over time, *not* smoking feels as natural to them as smoking did. Like them, you'll be more likely to live a longer, healthier life when you leave cigarettes behind.

How Nicotine Packs Its Punch

Nicotine affects your body in ways you might not expect. It's a greedy drug that wants to be everywhere at once. When you inhale smoke from a cigarette, nicotine goes deep into your lungs, where it's quickly absorbed into your bloodstream and carried to your heart, brain, liver, and spleen. It affects your heart and blood vessels, hormonal system, metabolism, and brain, among other body parts and functions. It also lowers your skin temperature and reduces blood flow in your legs and feet.

Feelin' Good. Nicotine gets to work right away. It reaches your brain only 7 seconds after you inhale cigarette smoke. This is the fastest delivery system of any drug—faster than marijuana, heroin, or cocaine. Then it fools your brain into feeling good by replacing other "feel-good" chemicals (like dopamine) that are naturally present in the brain. Tricky, huh? The first dose of nicotine makes you feel awake and alert, and later doses make you feel calm and relaxed.

The Body's Tolerance. When the body takes in nicotine regularly, it is affected by nicotine less and less. In other words, the body builds up a tolerance to nicotine and needs more and more nicotine to feel good. So a smoker craves cigarettes more often and smokes more often to get more nicotine in the blood. Eventually, a smoker reaches a certain nicotine level and then smokes

> ### ▶ ARE YOU ADDICTED TO NICOTINE?
>
> If you answer yes to any of the following questions, you may be physically addicted to nicotine.
>
> ❑ Do you smoke within 10 minutes of waking up each day?
>
> ❑ Would you still smoke if you were sick in bed most of the day?
>
> ❑ Do you have a hard time not smoking when you're in a nonsmoking area?
>
> ❑ When you've quit or tried to quit before, did you feel withdrawal symptoms or cravings?
>
> ❑ Have you ever smoked a cigarette when you didn't really want to smoke but felt like you *had* to?
>
> If you answered yes to 3 or more questions, you may have a strong addiction. Being aware of a physical addiction to nicotine will help you plan a way to quit.

as much as necessary to keep this level of nicotine in the bloodstream.

Part of the Problem: Withdrawal

In general, nicotine—the main addictive ingredient in tobacco—or cotinine (a nicotine by-product) stays in a regular smoker's body for 3 to 4 days after the person smokes. If someone has smoked regularly for at least a few weeks and then either stops using tobacco or really cuts down on the amount he or she smokes, this lowers the nicotine level in the person's blood so that the body begins missing its usual hit of nicotine. This can cause the person to automatically reach for a cigarette to raise the nicotine level in the blood. Without knowing it, the person is treating early withdrawal symptoms.

Stopping the use of any drug can cause side effects. If you have withdrawal symptoms after you quit smoking, it's because your body is getting used to going without the nicotine it has learned to lean on. So if you feel physically bad for a few days or weeks, it's because your body isn't getting the drug it wants. Withdrawal symptoms are temporary and are a good sign that you're leaving nicotine behind.

Constant Cravings. Cravings can be predictable—you may crave a cigarette when you first wake up, after your first cup of coffee, or whenever you're feeling angry or upset. When you have a craving, you *really* want to smoke. You may be a little distracted by wanting a smoke, or you may feel like you're going to scream if you don't smoke *right now*. You may feel like there's no way you can get through another moment without smoking.

The good news is this: You can. If you don't smoke, you'll get over your craving in a few minutes anyway, without caving in to nicotine's tricks. Cravings can be very powerful, but *cravings will pass whether you smoke a cigarette or not*. Realizing when and why cravings happen can help you talk yourself out of caving in to cravings when you quit smoking.

You May Feel Bad Because You're Being Good. Withdrawal symptoms make stopping smoking really difficult for a lot of people. But not everyone has withdrawal symptoms. Those who do might notice any of the following symptoms:

- depression
- feelings of frustration and anger
- irritability
- trouble sleeping
- difficulty concentrating
- restlessness
- headache

- tiredness
- increased appetite
- coughing
- cravings
- mood swings
- dizziness
- nervousness

Smokers who get withdrawal symptoms usually feel them within a few hours of the last cigarette smoked. They will feel the strongest symptoms 2 to 3 days later. Symptoms can last from a few days to several weeks. Smokers who have withdrawal symptoms cope with them for a while and end up feeling better than they ever did when they smoked. There are many ways you can learn to cope with these symptoms (see Chapter 3).

> ▶ **HOW TO QUIT**
>
> Studies have shown that these 5 steps will help you quit for good. You have the best chance of quitting if you adapt them to your quitting plan and follow them together:
>
> 1. Get ready.
> 2. Get support.
> 3. Learn new skills and behaviors.
> 4. Get medication and use it correctly.
> 5. Be prepared for relapse or difficult situations.

The Magic of Medications. Medications like nicotine replacement therapy, bupropion (Zyban), and vareniclinc (Chantix) can help decrease withdrawal symptoms (see Chapter 2). Nicotine replacement, like the patch or gum, provides your body with regular, small amounts of nicotine and gradually weans you off of it so you don't go through many withdrawal symptoms. Zyban is a prescription medication that helps reduce withdrawal symptoms and lessen cravings for many people. Chantix is a newer drug that helps block nicotine's effects and reduce withdrawal symptoms.

Leaning on Nicotine

Your need for tobacco is probably not only physical. If it were, you could stop smoking, work through any withdrawal symptoms, and never be tempted by cigarettes again. But for the vast majority of smokers, nicotine addiction is only one piece of the puzzle. People turn

> ▶ **WHY SMOKE?**
>
> Some people rely on cigarettes to help cope with anger, tension, sadness, or just out of habit. Many smokers use tobacco without stopping to think about the reasons why.

to cigarettes for many reasons: to adjust their moods, to cope with feelings, or just out of habit.

As you read this book and consider quitting smoking, you're working toward your goal of being a nonsmoker. Evaluating your smoking patterns will help you begin to figure out the best quitting plan for *you*.

Smoking is as much a mental addiction as it is a physical addiction. Some people reach for a cigarette to deal with anger or frustration, or they smoke when they feel happy. When these people quit smoking, they may crave cigarettes as soon as they begin to feel these emotions. They may not be comfortable without smoking to distract themselves from their emotions.

In Chapters 3 and 4, we'll help you determine how to get through the vulnerable moments without smoking.

Smoking "Triggers"

Can you count how many cigarettes you smoked today? Most smokers aren't sure how many cigarettes they regularly smoke. Over time, smokers become used to lighting a cigarette at certain times, when they feel a certain way, or when they're with certain people. You may also face regular triggers—situations, places, people, or feelings—that cause you to want to smoke.

When do you reach for a smoke? In the car? At breakfast? Waiting for the train? When you're bored, stressed, or angry? But you haven't *always* smoked while driving, after eating, when you wake up, or when you feel unhappy. You began by linking smoking to these situations and, along the way, the situation and the smoking became intertwined in your daily routine. Think about when you use cigarettes to get through your daily life. Do you see any patterns? Take the "Why Test" at the end of this chapter to discover your own reasons for reaching for a cigarette.

Certain strategies work best for people who rely on cigarettes for relaxation. Others will most help smokers who have become used to lighting up so they have something in their hands. In Chapter 2, we'll address ways to help you stop smoking and develop a quitting strategy that will work for you.

The Benefits of Your Doubts

In Chapter 3, we will show you specific ways to cope with some common fears about quitting smoking such as weight gain, stress, and being around friends and loved ones who smoke. We'll help you set up a simple, effective game plan to handle these challenges.

Many smokers also have general fears about quitting smoking. They may be afraid that it will simply be too hard and they'll "fail" or that it's too late to benefit from quitting. People can quit smoking—and improve their health—even when they've smoked 2 packs a day for 60 years. With a plan and support, anyone can quit.

"It's Too Hard to Quit"

Mark Twain said, "To cease smoking is the easiest thing I ever did. I ought to know, I've done it a thousand times." Maybe you've tried to quit before, too. It isn't easy for

> ▶ **FEAR OF FAILURE**
>
> Reports estimate that for nearly 70 percent of smokers, the possibility of failure stops them from trying to quit. You'll have the best chance for success if you set up a plan that's right for you and get all the support you can. Don't let fear of failure stop you from becoming a nonsmoker.

most people to give up tobacco, even though they have a lot of reasons to quit.

Let's be realistic. You won't forget about smoking forever just because you throw away your cigarettes and decide to quit. Quitting involves letting go of the habit, physical addiction, and psychological dependence on smoking.

"It's Too Late to Quit"

It's never too late to stop smoking. Whether you're 18 or 80 and whether you've smoked for a short time or a lifetime, quitting smoking will help you. It will improve your short-term and long-term health; fatten your wallet; stop your clothes, hair, car, house, and mouth from smelling like stale smoke; and help those around you stay healthy.

Your body is capable of repairing a lot of the damage caused by years of smoking. Within 20 minutes of your last cigarette, your body begins healing itself.

Quit Smoking for Good

Although everyone wants to quit on the first try, it takes most people more than one try to kick the habit for good. You may be one of those who can do it the first time. But if you're not, *don't give up.* (See Chapter 5 for more information.)

▶ MY MOST RECENT QUIT ATTEMPT

Reviewing your last quit attempt can help you learn how to improve your chances of quitting for good this time.

What worked?

- What kept me from smoking for a time? *(Thinking about your health status? Setting an example for your kids?)*

  _____

  _____

- How long did I go without smoking?

- Did I feel any improvements? *(In your breathing or stamina? Your wallet? The smell of your clothes?)*

  _____

  _____

What felt good about quitting?

- ❑ I felt healthier.
- ❑ I helped those around me be healthier.
- ❑ I saved money.
- ❑ Cigarettes didn't control me.
- ❑ I didn't smell like smoke.
- ❑ I set a good example.
- ❑ I was proud of myself.
- ❑ Other people were proud of me.
- ❑ Other good things:

  _____

  _____

  _____

  _____

(continued)

What was hard about quitting?

❑ Dealing with cravings for cigarettes

❑ Not knowing what to do with my hands

❑ Staying quit when others around me were smoking

❑ Not smoking when (*waking up? finishing a meal?*)

_____

❑ Not knowing what to do when (*angry, nervous, or upset?*)

❑ Other difficult things:

_____

_____

_____

What situation, emotion, or excuse led you to smoke again?

• Where was I?

• What was I doing?

• Who was I with?

• How was I feeling?

If you came across the same situation again, how could you deal with it without smoking?

I could . . .

_____

_____

_____

_____

(continued)

Throughout this book we'll outline how you can cope with situations like the one in which you smoked again — and the times and places that make you regularly want to smoke now. *You can handle each of them* — without smoking.

If You've Tried to Quit Before

You may wonder why this attempt to quit might be any different. Having tried to quit before can actually help you quit this time.

About 70 percent of smokers say they would like to quit, and about 40 percent of smokers actually try to quit each year. Each time you try to quit, you learn what works for you and what doesn't. So you have an advantage this time around if you've tried to stop smoking before. Think of the last time as a trial run.

Call It Quits: Why Do You Want to Quit?

As you consider committing to quit, think about some "flashbulb" reminders. These will become part of "My Quitting Reminders"—quick, powerful reminders that can stop you in your tracks when you have the impulse to smoke.

Post your list of reasons to quit and the quitting reminders you developed everywhere you used to smoke so you see them: the car dashboard, your desk, your bedside table, and the kitchen. Make a deal with yourself that if you feel the urge to smoke, you'll look at your nearby reminders. Promise yourself that you'll stop and reflect on each reason you wrote down when you started this journey. The urge to smoke will probably have lessened by the time you finish reading. Refer

▶ MY QUITTING REMINDERS

Think about your unique reasons for wanting to stop smoking. What themes can you see? Health? Money? Control? Other things?

Think about what's important to you as you get ready to commit to quit. What is it about smoking that creates these feelings?

- Frustration? *(Not being able to do the things you want to?)*

  _____

- Anger? *(The money you spend on cigarettes?)*

  _____

- Fatigue? *(The stress of having cigarettes control your life?)*

  _____

- Fear? *(The effects of smoking on your health?)*

  _____

What might have the power to remind you of your reasons to quit? Write down in large print or tape each one on a piece of paper.

- One word *("cancer"? "health"? "future"? "$$$"? your children's names?)*:

  _____

- One sentence *("I want to stop wasting my money"? "Smoking controls my life"? "I want to live to be 85"? "I don't want to be a smoker anymore"?)*:

  _____

  _____

(continued)

- One picture *(a photo of grandchildren? a picture of blackened lungs? a photo of a vacation spot where you want to go with the money you would have spent on cigarettes?)*:

_____

What will help you forget about smoking as an option? Your quitting reminders will help you remember why you wanted to stop smoking in the first place.

to "My Quitting Reminders" as many times a day as you need to keep yourself from smoking.

Commit to Quit

Quitting smoking is a lot like losing weight. It takes a strong commitment over time to succeed. That's why only you can make the decision to quit smoking. Other people may want you to quit, but the real commitment to quit must come from you.

You're moving right along on your path to quitting smoking! If you are serious about quitting smoking and feel that you'll be ready to quit within the next month, begin making a quitting plan. The first step is scheduling a Quit Day—the day you'll quit smoking.

Make It Official: Schedule Your Quit Day

Once you've decided to quit, make it official by picking a Quit Day. Choose a day in the next month when you don't expect to be under much pressure or facing a big challenge. Life is full of everyday stresses, but only a major change in your life or a tragedy should make you consider putting off your Quit Day.

> ▶ **ARE YOU READY TO COMMIT TO QUIT?**
>
> Do you feel ready to take the next step? Find out by answering the following questions:
>
> ❑ Do you believe that you can make an honest attempt at quitting smoking?
>
> ❑ Do you think that the benefits of quitting outweigh the benefits of continuing to smoke?
>
> ❑ Do you know of someone who has had health problems as a result of smoking?
>
> ❑ Do you think you could get a smoking-related disease, and does this worry you?
>
> Answering yes to these questions means you may be ready to make a serious attempt to quit.

You might even want to choose a special day like your birthday, your anniversary, or the Great American Smokeout®. Each November, about 17 million people try to quit for at least a day during the American Cancer Society's Great American Smokeout. Of these quitters, more than 4 million still aren't smoking after 3 months.

Once you've decided on a date, write it down here.

This is my Quit Day: _____

Make a strong, personal commitment to quit on this day.

• Write your Quit Day on your calendar and in this book to cement its "official" status in your mind.

- Tell friends and family about it so you'll be less likely to put it off.

- Consider your Quit Day to be sacred, and don't let anything change it.

Congratulations! You're on your way! In the next chapter we'll explore choices of how to quit and help you figure out which of them are best suited to your smoking patterns. That'll help you kick butts for good.

Why Do You Smoke?

This quiz can help you understand why you smoke. Once you understand the reasons why you smoke, you'll be able to create a unique plan for quitting smoking.

▶ **THE "WHY TEST"**

Next to the following statements, mark the number that best describes your own experience. (5 = Always, 4 = Most of the time, 3 = Once in a while, 2 = Rarely, 1 = Never)

_____ **A.** I smoke to keep myself from slowing down.

_____ **B.** Handling a cigarette is part of the enjoyment of smoking it.

_____ **C.** Smoking is pleasant and relaxing.

_____ **D.** I light up a cigarette when I feel angry about something.

_____ **E.** When I am out of cigarettes, it's near-torture until I can get more.

_____ **F.** I smoke automatically, without even being aware of it.

(continued)

_____ **G.** I smoke when people around me are smoking.

_____ **H.** I smoke to perk myself up.

_____ **I.** Part of my enjoyment of smoking is preparing to light up.

_____ **J.** I get pleasure from smoking.

_____ **K.** When I feel uncomfortable or upset, I light up a cigarette.

_____ **L.** When I am not smoking a cigarette, I'm very much aware of the fact.

_____ **M.** I often light up a cigarette when one is still burning in the ashtray.

_____ **N.** I smoke cigarettes with friends when I am having a good time.

_____ **O.** When I smoke, part of the enjoyment is watching the smoke as I exhale.

_____ **P.** I want a cigarette most often when I am comfortable and relaxed.

_____ **Q.** I smoke when I am "blue" and want to take my mind off of what is bothering me.

_____ **R.** I get a real hunger for a cigarette when I haven't had one in a while.

_____ **S.** I've found a cigarette in my mouth and haven't remembered it was there.

_____ **T.** I always smoke when I am out with friends at a party, bar, etc.

_____ **U.** I always smoke cigarettes to get a lift.

(continued)

Now Score Yourself

Step 1: Transfer the numbers from the quiz to the scorecard that follows by matching up the letters. For example, take the number you wrote for question A on the quiz and enter it on line A of the scorecard.

Step 2: Add each set of 3 scores on the scorecard to get the total for each different category. For example, find your score on the "Stimulation" category; add together the score for questions A, H, and U.

The score for each category can range from a low of 3 to a high of 15. A score of 11 or above on any set is high and means that your smoking is probably influenced by that category. A score of 7 or below is low and means that this category is not a primary source of satisfaction to you when you smoke.

"Why Test" scorecard

"It stimulates me." You feel that smoking gives you energy and keeps you going. Think about alternative ways to boost your energy, such as brisk walking or jogging.

_____ A.   _____ H.   _____ U.

_____ "Stimulation" TOTAL

"I want something in my hand." There are a lot of things you can do with your hands without lighting up a cigarette. Try doodling with a pencil or playing with putty or a fake cigarette.

_____ B.   _____ I.   _____ O.

_____ "Handling" TOTAL

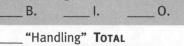

(continued)

"It feels good." You get a lot of physical pleasure from smoking. Various forms of exercise or other activities can be effective alternatives.

_____ C.   _____ J.   _____ P.

_____ **"Pleasure/Relaxation" TOTAL**

"It's a crutch." It can be tough to stop smoking if you find cigarettes comforting in times of stress, but there are many better ways to deal with stress.

_____ D.   _____ K.   _____ Q.

_____ **"Crutch/Tension" TOTAL**

"I'm hooked." In addition to having a psychological addiction to smoking, you may also be physically addicted to nicotine. It's a hard addiction to break, but it can be done. Talk with your doctor about using nicotine replacement (the gum, patch, inhaler, or nasal spray) to control your withdrawal symptoms.

_____ E.   _____ L.   _____ R.

_____ **"Craving/Addiction" TOTAL**

"It's part of my routine." If cigarettes are merely part of your routine, stopping should be relatively easy. One key to success is being aware of every cigarette you smoke. Keeping a smoking diary is a good way to do this.

_____ F.   _____ M.   _____ S.

_____ **"Habit" TOTAL**

"I'm a social smoker." You smoke when people around you are smoking and when you are offered

(continued)

cigarettes. It is important for you to avoid these situations until you are confident about being a nonsmoker. If you cannot avoid a situation in which others are smoking, remind them that you are a nonsmoker.

_____ G.   _____ N.   _____ T.

_____ "Social Smoker" **TOTAL**

Now how do I quit?

We hope this quiz has provided some insight into the reasons why you smoke. This information may be used to help you stop smoking. Talk to your doctor about how to stop and how to stay tobacco free.

Reprinted with permission from "Smoking: 'Why Do I Smoke?' Quiz," January 2008, http://familydoctor.org/296.xml.

How to Quit: It's Up to You

THERE'S NO "RIGHT" WAY to quit smoking. Things that help you may seem silly to others, and those that help other people may not help you. Don't be afraid to try something new or something you hadn't planned to help you quit. The best way to quit is to use the method that works for you.

Remember how powerful nicotine is? Well, it isn't always easy to drop the smoking habit, and most people need some sort of help as they quit. Using support doesn't mean that you're weak or more addicted than most. It just shows that you're smart to use all the resources you can to increase your chances of success.

Nicotine replacement therapy (the patch, gum, nasal spray, lozenge, and inhaler) and other medications safely help a lot of smokers quit, and organized support from other people increases success rates even more.

Before your Quit Day, you can prepare for success by creating a personal plan to help you quit and thinking about the support you'll rely on as you quit. That's what we'll help you do here.

Talk to the Professionals

Ask your doctor about current information, advice, and suggestions for quitting tobacco use. You may choose to stop smoking without using prescription medicine. However, for the following reasons, it's a good idea to check with a health care professional before you quit:

- He or she can review your personal health history and offer advice and information about which medications might be right for you.

- He or she can give you tips on quitting and offer follow-up support.

- Health care professionals are usually the first ones to learn about new, effective ways of quitting. They can also help steer you away from unproven or disproven stop-smoking methods.

Don't Chicken Out: Go Cold Turkey

Most smokers quit "cold turkey." That is, they smoke until their Quit Day and then stop all at once. This is the fastest way to quit and, for most people, the most successful way to quit. Gradually cutting down the number of cigarettes you smoke each day usually doesn't work because a lot of people have a hard time giving up those last few cigarettes.

Never Fear, Medications Are Here

Stop-smoking medications can more or less double your chances of quitting for good. Evidence has shown, for example, that nicotine replacement therapies boost smoking cessation rates and combining nicotine replacement therapy with bupropion (Zyban, a non-nicotine prescription medication) may even be more effective.*

▶ TALK TO A HEALTH CARE PROFESSIONAL

Before your Quit Day, set up an appointment to talk with a health care professional. Talk to your doctor about the details of your health, smoking patterns, past quit attempts, and any concerns you may have. As your prepare for your appointment, consider the following issues:

I want you to be aware of my health conditions (*including pregnancy if applicable, and mention any medications you are currently taking*):

_____

_____

These are some things that worked and others that didn't during my past quit attempts:

_____

_____

Here are my concerns about medication side effects and nicotine withdrawal:

_____

_____

(*continued*)

*__Source:__ Jorenby DE, Leischow SJ, Nides MA, Rennard SI, Johnston JA, Hughes AR, Smith SS, Muramoto ML, Daughton DM, Doan K, Fiore MC, Baker TB. A controlled trial of sustained-release bupropion, a nicotine patch, or both for smoking cessation. *N Engl J Med*. 1999;340:685–691.

What do I do if I experience side effects?

_____

_____

_____

How can I benefit from nicotine replacement, bupropion, or varenicline, considering my smoking patterns?_____

_____

_____

Note: If you are a very heavy smoker or a very light smoker, you may need to work with your doctor to ensure that your therapy fits your situation. If you don't use enough nicotine replacement, for example, you may experience withdrawal symptoms that make you want to start smoking again. If you use too much, you could make yourself sick or seriously ill.

Medications treat the physical addiction to nicotine. They cut down on withdrawal symptoms, but they don't magically stop you from being faced with your triggers to smoke. That's why it works best to combine stop-smoking medications with other types of support. Combining them with a stop-smoking program that helps change behavior can increase your chances of successfully quitting smoking.

Using a medication can help *anyone* who is trying to quit. Nicotine replacement therapy and bupropion are safe for most people. Varenicline is an option for others. If you're pregnant or trying to become pregnant, breastfeeding, under age 18, smoking fewer than 10 cigarettes per day, or have a medical condition, talk to your doctor or other health care provider before taking medications. See also "Is nicotine replacement safe for everyone?" on page 40.

Use It: Nicotine Replacement Therapy

Using nicotine replacement therapy instead of smoking allows your body to get a low dose of the nicotine it's used to without the poisons and tar in cigarettes and cigarette smoke. This temporary substitute helps reduce withdrawal symptoms, in turn helping you reduce cravings and adapt to living your daily life without smoking.

▶ A WINNING COMBINATION?

Studies show that combining the nicotine patch with shorter-acting products such as the gum, lozenge, nasal spray, or inhaler may work better than using a patch alone.* The idea is to get a steady dose of nicotine with the patch and to use one of the shorter-acting products when you have strong cravings. For example, in studies that have combined the nicotine patch and nicotine gum, smokers used the nicotine patches routinely, then used the nicotine gum only when they had a craving.

*Sources: Blondal T, Gudmundsson LJ, Olafsdottir I, Gustavsson G, Westin A. Nicotine nasal spray with nicotine patch for smoking cessation: randomized trial with six year follow up. *BMJ.* 1999;318:285–289.

Bohadana A, Nilsson F, Rasmussen T, Martinet Y. Nicotine inhaler and nicotine patch as a combination therapy for smoking cessation: A randomized, double-blind, placebo-controlled trial. *Arch Intern Med.* 2000;160:3128–3134.

Stead LF, Perera R, Bullen C, Mant D, Lancaster T. Nicotine replacement therapy for smoking cessation. *Cochrane Database of Systematic Reviews.* 2008, Issue 1. Art. No.: CD000146. DOI: 10.1002/14651858. DC000146.pub3.

Note: The combined use of nicotine replacement products has not yet been approved by the U.S. Food and Drug Administration (FDA). Therefore, if you are considering the option of using more than one nicotine replacement product, talk it over with your doctor first.

Stick It: The Nicotine Patch. Also known as nicotine transdermal systems, nicotine patches stick to the skin and provide a constant, measured dose of nicotine through the skin. Read the instructions and safety precautions on the package insert before using the patch. The patch is available over the counter, without a prescription.

Some advantages of the nicotine patch include the following:

- It's easy to use—you only have to remember to replace the patch each day.

- The constant nicotine dosage helps keep you from feeling cravings.

The nicotine in the patch reaches the bloodstream over several hours and continues entering the bloodstream several hours after the patch is removed, so don't smoke within 12 hours of removing the patch.

Several types and strengths of the patch are available. If you use the step-down method, the patches you use contain less and less nicotine so you'll be weaned off nicotine without experiencing withdrawal symptoms.

■ **possible side effects:** A mild itching, burning, or tingling at the site of the patch when it is first applied is normal, but should go away within an hour. Try a different brand of patch if your skin continues to be irritated.

The 24-hour patch almost always causes strange effects, including vivid, colorful dreams and difficulty sleeping. If sleep problems don't stop within 3 or 4 days, try switching to a 16-hour patch.

If any side effects are severe or continue, talk to your doctor about using a lower-dose patch or trying a different form of nicotine replacement.

Chew and Park It: Nicotine Gum. Nicotine gum (nicotine polacrilex) is a fast-acting form of nicotine replacement. For best results, follow the instructions on the package insert. Nicotine gum can be bought over the counter.

Some advantages of nicotine gum include the following:

- It allows you to control when you receive a nicotine dose.

- The gum may be better than the patch for people with sensitive skin.

- The gum can be chewed as needed or on a fixed schedule during the day.

You don't constantly chew nicotine gum like you do other gum. Chew nicotine gum slowly until you notice a peppery taste. Then "park" it against the cheek, chewing it and parking it off and on for about 20 to 30 minutes. Food and drink can affect how well the nicotine is absorbed, so avoid acidic foods and drinks like coffee, juice, and soft drinks for at least 15 minutes before using the gum and while using the gum.

Chewing the gum releases nicotine, which is absorbed through the lining of the mouth. The nicotine in the gum takes a few minutes to reach the brain, so the nicotine "rush" is less intense than with a cigarette. The higher dose of nicotine gum that is available may help heavier smokers.

Nicotine gum may not be the right choice for those with temporomandibular joint disease (TMJ) or for those with dentures or other vulnerable dental work.

■ **possible side effects:** Some possible side effects of nicotine gum include the following: bad taste, throat irritation, mouth ulcers, hiccups, nausea, jaw discomfort, and racing heartbeat. Talk to your health care professional if you experience ongoing side effects while using nicotine gum.

Follow Your Nose: Nicotine Nasal Spray. Nicotine nasal spray quickly sends nicotine to the bloodstream through the nose. Read the package instructions and safety precautions before using. It is available by prescription only.

Some advantages of nicotine nasal spray include the following:

- It gives immediate relief of withdrawal symptoms.

- It is easy to use.

- Its quick "rush" of nicotine may especially help heavily addicted smokers.

Follow instructions closely to make sure you get the amount of nasal spray you need to fight withdrawal symptoms. If you have asthma, allergies, nasal polyps, or sinus problems, your health care professional may suggest a different form of nicotine replacement.

■ **possible side effects:** The most common side effects last about 1 to 2 weeks and can include the following: nasal irritation, runny nose, watery eyes, sneezing, throat irritation, and coughing. Talk to your health care professional if you experience ongoing side effects while using nicotine nasal spray.

Take a Breath: The Nicotine Inhaler. The nicotine inhaler is a plastic tube about the size of a cigarette with a nicotine cartridge inside. Read the instructions and safety precautions on the package insert before using the inhaler. The nicotine inhaler is available by prescription.

Some advantages of the nicotine inhaler include the following:

- You can control the amount of nicotine you get when you have an urge to smoke.

- You may be able to satisfy a craving for a hand-to-mouth action by using the nicotine inhaler.

When you puff on the inhaler, the cartridge delivers a nicotine vapor to the mouth. One inhaler cartridge contains about the same amount of nicotine found in two cigarettes.

■ **possible side effects:** Side effects from the inhaler can include coughing or mouth or throat irritation. You may also have an upset stomach. These symptoms should decrease over time. If you have a disease like asthma that causes airway spasms, talk to your doctor about whether the nicotine inhaler is right for you. Talk to your health care professional if you have ongoing side effects while using the nicotine inhaler.

Try a Lozenge: Nicotine Lozenges. Nicotine-containing lozenges as an over-the-counter aid to stop smoking are the newest form of nicotine replacement therapy on the market. As with nicotine gum, lozenges are available in 2 strengths. Smokers choose their dose based on how long after waking up they normally have their first cigarette.

You should stop all smoking when you start using lozenges. Do not eat or drink for 15 minutes after taking a lozenge. (Some drinks can reduce how well the lozenge works.) Suck on the lozenge until it is fully dissolved—about 20 to 30 minutes. Do not bite or chew it like hard candy, and do not swallow it. Do not use more than 20 lozenges per day. Lozenges should be used for no more than 12 weeks.

Some advantages of the lozenge include the following:

- It allows you to control when you need a nicotine dose.

- It delivers nicotine to the brain in minutes, rather than in hours (as with the patch).

- It requires little effort to use and may be good for those who want to be inconspicuous about their quitting.

■ **possible side effects:** Possible side effects of the nicotine lozenge include the following: soreness of the teeth and gums, indigestion, and irritated throat. These side effects are usually short-lived and are less likely with use as directed. The lozenge should not be bitten into or chewed, as this will cause more nicotine to be swallowed quickly and result in indigestion and/ or heartburn. Lozenge users may also have trouble sleeping, nausea, hiccups, coughing, headache, and flatulence (gas).

Which Type of Nicotine Replacement May Be Right for You?

There's no evidence that any one type of nicotine replacement therapy is any better than another. When choosing a type of nicotine replacement therapy, think about which method will best fit your lifestyle and pattern of smoking. Do you want/need something to chew or to occupy your hands? Or are you looking for once-a-day convenience?

Consider the following important points:

- Nicotine gums, lozenges, and inhalers are substitutes you can put in your mouth that allow you to control your dosage to help keep cravings under control.

- Nicotine nasal spray works very quickly when you need it.

- Nicotine inhalers allow you to mimic the use of cigarettes by puffing and holding the inhaler.

- Nicotine patches are convenient and only have to be applied once a day.

- Both inhalers and nasal sprays require a doctor's prescription.

- Some people may not be able to use patches, inhalers, or nasal sprays because of allergies or other conditions.

- Nicotine gums and lozenges are generally sugar-free, but if you are diabetic and have any doubts, check with the manufacturer.

Whatever type of nicotine replacement therapy you select, always treat it with respect as you would other medications. Read the product inserts and carefully follow package directions. Package inserts describe how to use each product and also address special issues and possible side effects. Many companies that make nicotine replacement systems offer support, tips, and safety information on their Web sites.

All nicotine replacement therapies produce side effects, but they're rarely severe enough that you should stop using the products. Depending on how much you smoked, you may still experience some withdrawal symptoms when you use nicotine replacement. Many people who have withdrawal symptoms while using nicotine

> ### ▶ CANDY-COATING NICOTINE
>
> Some pharmacies in the United States sell products called "nicotine lollipops" and "nicotine lip balm," which they promote as helpful for people who are quitting smoking. These products often contain a product called nicotine salicylate, a form of nicotine that is not approved by the FDA for use in quitting smoking. The FDA has warned those who sell nicotine lollipops and lip balm in pharmacies and on the Internet that the products are illegal.
>
> Other similar stop-smoking products may not use nicotine salicylate and may be legal. All of these products pose a risk to children because they often look like candy.

replacement therapy are using too little of the medication for their specific needs. Talk to your health care provider if your craving for cigarettes continues, if you feel irritable, or if you have a hard time concentrating.

Is nicotine replacement safe for everyone? Not everyone can use nicotine replacement. The following people should get medical advice before using any kind of nicotine replacement therapy:

- people with heart or circulatory diseases
- people with high blood pressure
- pregnant women
- women who are breastfeeding
- people under the age of 18

> **▶ NO SMOKING!**
>
> Do *not* use nicotine replacement if you plan to keep smoking or use another tobacco product. It is possible to get an overdose of nicotine. Signs of overdose include headaches, dizziness, upset stomach, vomiting, diarrhea, mental confusion, weakness, or fainting.

If you take any medications, especially drugs for asthma or depression, talk to your doctor. Your medication dose may need to be adjusted because, with or without nicotine replacement, the body changes when you stop smoking.

Keep nicotine replacement products, including those that have been used and thrown away, out of reach of children and pets. Even very small amounts of nicotine can make them seriously ill.

Will I be able to quit using nicotine replacement? Some people worry that they'll become dependent on the small amounts of nicotine in the various forms of nicotine replacement therapy. This rarely happens. Most of these products are meant to be used for 2 to 3 months. To help you gradually taper off the nicotine, you use smaller doses of these products over time.

Prescription Medications Can Help

Research has shown that using a smoking cessation drug, such as bupropion (Zyban), varenicline (Chantix), or the nicotine patch, gum, nasal spray, inhaler, or lozenge, can double your chances of successfully quitting.

- **Bupropion** is a non-nicotine, prescription medicine that helps reduce cravings.

- **Varenicline** is a drug that helps lessen nicotine withdrawal symptoms and lowers the feelings of pleasure people get from smoking.

- **Nicotine replacement products** can help with uncomfortable physical withdrawal symptoms, giving you the chance to concentrate on changing the "habit" or routine of smoking.

Talk to your doctor or health care provider about a strategy that will work for you. Depending on your smoking habits and previous attempts to quit, your doctor may recommend using one or more of these products. It is likely, though, that your doctor will not recommend using varenicline with nicotine replacement products. In early testing, adding a nicotine replacement drug to varenicline resulted in side effects that were more unpleasant than those associated with varenicline alone.*

If you are having a lot of trouble quitting, your doctor might prescribe bupropion to be used with nicotine replacement therapy. It will depend on your health, what other medicines you are taking, and the safety of using both at the same time.

Bupropion (Zyban)

Bupropion, a prescription drug used to treat depression, was also the first medical stop-smoking aid that did not contain nicotine. It's not clear exactly how bupropion helps smokers quit, but some people think it affects the chemicals in the brain related to nicotine cravings.

*Source: Pfizer Labs (Division of Pfizer Inc.). Chantix® (varenicline) tablets: full prescribing information. Pfizer Web site. http://media.pfizer .com/files/products/uspi_chantix.pdf. Accessed March 3, 2010.

Some advantages of bupropion include the following*:

- Bupropion can help reduce weight gain.

- Bupropion is safe to use with nicotine replacement therapy.

- Smokers begin taking bupropion before they quit smoking, which lessens cravings by getting the body ready before taking away nicotine.

- People who haven't been helped by nicotine replacement therapies may have success with bupropion.

Bupropion is easy to use. You should begin taking it 1 to 2 weeks before you quit smoking to make sure it reaches the right levels in your body to be effective; then you continue taking it for at least 7 to 12 weeks after you quit. It is taken regularly to manage cravings: once in the morning and once in the late afternoon. Evidence suggests that it may be more effective to combine nicotine replacement therapy with bupropion than to use either one on its own. See the "Be Careful" section on the next page for more information.

■ **possible side effects:** Some common side effects from bupropion are dry mouth, difficulty sleeping, restlessness, anxiety, shakiness, headaches, and a rash. As many as 3 in 1,000 people taking bupropion

*__Sources:__ Hurt RD, Sachs DPL, Glover ED, Offord KP, Johnston JA, Dale LC, Khayrallah MA, Schroeder DR, Glover PN, Sullivan CR, Croghan IT, Sullivan PM. A comparison of sustained-release bupropion and placebo for smoking cessation. *N Engl J Med.* 1997;337:1195–1202.

Jorenby DE, Leischow SJ, Nides MA, Rennard SI, Johnston JA, Hughes AR, Smith SS, Muramoto ML, Daughton DM, Doan K, Fiore MC, Baker TB. A controlled trial of sustained-release bupropion, a nicotine patch, or both for smoking cessation. *N Engl J Med.* 1999;340:685–691.

▶ **BE CAREFUL**

- Do not take bupropion if you have a history of seizures; anorexia or bulimia (eating disorders); heavy alcohol or drug use; bipolar (manic-depressive) illness; or head trauma.

- Do not take bupropion with other medications containing bupropion or monoamine oxidase (MAO) inhibitors (drugs that treat mood disorders).

- Tell your doctor if you are taking any vitamins or herbs, as well as any of the following drugs that may result in serious side effects when combined with bupropion: Tegretol, cimetidine, phenobarbitol, Dilantin, MAO inhibitors, L-dopa or other seizure medicines, other antidepressants, heart rhythm drugs, drugs for serious mental illness, or HIV treatment drugs.

- Tell your doctor if you have liver, heart, or kidney disease; if you have high blood pressure, lung disease, diabetes, gout, or infections; if you are pregnant or breastfeeding; or if you've recently had a heart attack or bouts of chest pain.

- Don't drink alcohol while taking bupropion.

may have an allergic reaction—like itching, rash, and hives—serious enough for them to need medical attention. Some people may feel more agitated, anxious, and restless or have trouble sleeping when they begin taking this drug. If these side effects don't go away after a few days, call your health care provider.

Varenicline (Chantix)

Varenicline (Chantix) is a newer prescription medicine specifically developed to help people stop smoking. Varenicline interferes with nicotine receptors in the brain, resulting in 2 effects: it lessens the pleasurable physical effects a person gets from smoking, and it reduces the symptoms of nicotine withdrawal.

Several studies have shown that varenicline can more than double the chances of quitting smoking. Some studies have also found it may work better than bupropion, at least in the short term.*

Varenicline is taken in pill form, beginning with a small dose of 0.5 mg each day. The daily dose is increased over the first 8 days it is taken. For people who have problems with the higher dose, a lower dose may be used during the quit effort. Varenicline is given for 12 weeks, but people who quit during that time may get another 12 weeks of treatment to boost their chance of quitting.

■ **possible side effects:** Some common side effects from varenicline are headaches, nausea, vomiting, trouble sleeping, unusual dreams, flatulence (gas), and changes in taste. There have also been more recent reports of depressed mood, thoughts of suicide, attempted suicide, and changes in behavior in people taking varenicline. People who have these problems should contact

*Sources: Gonzales D, Rennard SI, Nides M, Oncken C, Azoulay S, Billing CB, Watsky EJ, Gong J, Williams KE, Reeves KR, for the Varenicline Phase 3 Study Group. Varenicline, an α4β2 nicotinic acetylcholine receptor partial agonist, vs sustained-release bupropion and placebo for smoking cessation. A randomized controlled trial. *JAMA.* 2006;296:47–55.

U.S. Food and Drug Administration (2006). FDA approves novel medication for smoking cessation. *FDA News.* U.S Food and Drug Administration Web site. http://www.fda.gov/NewsEvents/Newsroom/Press Announcements/2006/ucm108651.htm. Accessed March 3, 2010.

their doctors right away. Although these side effects may happen, varenicline is usually well tolerated.

Since varenicline is a newer drug, research has not been done to find out whether it is safe to use along with nicotine replacement therapy products. But the company that makes varenicline noted that people who used the drug along with nicotine replacement therapy had more side effects such as nausea and headaches.

Other Drugs Not FDA Approved for Helping Smokers Quit

Other drugs have shown promise in research studies for smokers who are trying to quit but cannot use any of the FDA-approved stop-smoking drugs and for smokers who have been unable to quit smoking with use of the FDA-approved drugs. The other drugs are recommended by the Agency for Healthcare Research and Quality (AHRQ) to help people quit smoking, but have not been approved by the FDA for this purpose and are used "off-label."

Note: The other drugs are available only with a prescription and are not recommended for pregnant smokers, teens, or people who smoke less than 10 cigarettes per day.

Nortriptyline

Nortriptyline is an older antidepressant drug. When used in groups of smokers, it has been found to double their chances of success in quitting smoking.* It is started 10 to 28 days before you stop smoking to allow it to reach a stable level in the body.

*__Sources:__ Hughes JR, Stead LF, Lancaster T. Nortriptyline for smoking cessation: a review. *Nicotine Tob Res*. 2005;7(4):491–499.
Hughes JR, Stead LF, Lancaster T. Antidepressants for smoking cessation. *Cochrane Database Syst Rev*. 2007;(1):CD000031.

■ **possible side effects:** Some common side effects from nortriptyline include fast heart rate, blurred vision, trouble urinating, dry mouth, constipation, weight gain or loss, and low blood pressure upon standing. The drug can impair one's ability to drive or operate machinery.

There are certain drugs that cannot be used along with nortriptyline. Be sure your doctor and pharmacist know exactly what you are taking before you start this medication. Also, be sure you know how to take it and how to taper it down when you are ready to stop. The dose of nortriptyline must be gradually lowered, since the drug cannot be stopped suddenly without the possibility of serious effects. The drug must be used with caution in people with heart disease.

Clonidine

Clonidine is an older drug that is FDA approved for the treatment of high blood pressure. When used for smoking cessation, it can be taken in the form of a pill, twice a day, or as a skin patch, applied once a week. In one study of heavy smokers who had failed in previous quit attempts, the group treated with clonidine was twice as likely to succeed in quitting smoking as the control group (which was given a placebo) at the end of 4 weeks.*

■ **possible side effects:** The most common side effects of clonidine are constipation, dizziness, drowsiness, dry mouth, and unusual tiredness or weakness. There are rarely more severe side effects, such as allergic

---

*Source: Glassman AH, Stetner F, Walsh BT, Raizman PS, Fleiss JL, Cooper TB, Covey LS. Heavy smokers, smoking cessation, and clonidine. Results of a double-blind, randomized trial. *JAMA.* 1988;259(19):2863–2866.

reactions, slow heart rate, and very high or very low blood pressure. The drug can impair one's ability to drive or operate machinery.

Be sure your doctor and pharmacist know exactly what you are taking before you start this medicine. Your doctor may want to watch your blood pressure while you are on this drug.

Clonidine can be started up to 3 days before you quit smoking, but it can also be started the day you quit. Like nortriptyline, it should not be stopped suddenly. The dose must be lowered over a period of 2 to 4 days to prevent a rapid increase in blood pressure, agitation, confusion, or tremors.

Other Methods of Quitting

Other tools may also help some people, although there is no strong evidence they can improve your chances of quitting.

Hypnosis

The methods of hypnosis vary, so it is difficult to study this method as a way to stop smoking. For the most part, reviews that looked at studies of hypnosis to help people quit smoking have not supported it as a quitting method that works. Still, some people find it useful. If you are interested in trying it, ask your doctor if he or she can recommend a good hypnotherapist.

Acupuncture

Although acupuncture has been used to quit smoking, there is little evidence to show that it works. Acupuncture for smoking is usually done on certain parts of the ears. Although there is a very weak suggestion that acupuncture might lower the desire to smoke, there still is no solid evidence that it is truly effective as a smoking cessation tool. For a list of local physician acupuncturists, contact the American Academy of Medical Acupuncture at 323-937-5514 or visit their Web site at www.medical acupuncture.org.

Low-level Laser Therapy

Also called cold laser therapy, low-level laser therapy is related to acupuncture. Cold lasers are sometimes used for acupuncture in place of needles to stimulate the body's acupoints. The treatment is supposed to relax the smoker and release endorphins (pain relief substances that are made naturally by the body) to mimic the effects of nicotine in the brain, or balance the body's energy to relieve the addiction. Despite claims of success by some cold laser therapy providers, there is no scientific evidence to show that this is an effective method of helping people stop smoking.

Filters

Filters that reduce tar and nicotine in cigarettes are generally not effective. Studies have shown that smokers who use filters actually tend to smoke more.

Smoking Deterrents

Other methods have been used to help stop smoking, such as over-the-counter products that change the taste of tobacco, stop-smoking diets that curb nicotine cravings, and combinations of vitamins. At this time, there is little scientific evidence that these efforts work.

Herbs and Supplements

There is little scientific evidence to support the use of homeopathic aids and herbal supplements as stop-smoking methods. Because they are marketed as dietary supplements (as opposed to drugs), they don't need FDA approval to be sold. The manufacturers don't have to prove they're effective or even safe. Be skeptical when any product claims it can help you stop smoking. No dietary supplement has been proven to effectively help people quit smoking. Most of these supplements are combinations of herbal preparations but do not contain nicotine. They have no proven track record of helping people stop smoking.

Atropine and Scopolamine Combination Therapy

A few smoking cessation clinics offer a program using the drugs atropine and scopolamine given as injections, sometimes along with other drugs, to help reduce nicotine withdrawal symptoms. These drugs block the action of acetylcholine, a signal transmitter in the nervous system. Called anticholinergics, they are more often prescribed for other reasons, such as digestive problems, motion sickness, or Parkinson's disease. People who are pregnant or have heart problems, glaucoma, or uncontrolled high blood pressure are not allowed to take part in these programs.

The treatment usually involves shots given in the clinic on one day, then a few weeks of pills and wearing patches behind the ear. Other drugs may be needed to help with side effects. Side effects of this treatment can include dizziness, constipation, dry mouth, changes in the sense of taste and smell, problems urinating, and blurry vision.

Some clinics claim high success rates, but the available published scientific research does not back up these claims. Both atropine and scopolamine are FDA-approved for other uses and have not been formally studied or approved for use in quitting smoking. Before going into such a program, you may want to ask the clinic about long-term success rates (up to a year). These medicines are directed only at the physical aspect of quitting, so you may also want to find out if the program includes counseling or other methods aimed at the psychological aspects of quitting.

Other Nicotine and Tobacco Products Not Reviewed or Approved by the FDA

Tobacco Lozenges and Pouches

Lozenges that contain tobacco (Ariva, Interval) and small pouches of tobacco (Revel, Exalt) are being sold as other ways for smokers to get nicotine in places where smoking is not allowed. The FDA has ruled that these are types of oral tobacco products much like snuff and chew and are not smoking cessation aids. This means that the FDA does not have authority over them. Unlike scientifically proven treatments with known effects, such as nicotine replacement products, antidepressants, nicotine receptor blockers, or behavioral therapy, these oral tobacco products have never been rigorously tested to see if they can help people quit using tobacco.

We know that oral tobacco products such as snuff and chewing tobacco contain carcinogens. These products cause mouth cancer and gum disease. They also destroy the bone sockets around teeth and can cause teeth to fall out. There are studies showing potential harmful effects on the heart and circulation, as well as increased risk of other cancers. They also cause bad breath and stain the teeth.

Electronic Cigarettes

In 2004, a Chinese company started making a refillable "cigarette" that had a battery and an electronic chip in it. It is designed to look like a cigarette, right down to the glowing tip. When the smoker puffs on it, the system delivers a mist of liquid, flavorings, and nicotine that looks something like smoke. The smoker inhales it like cigarette smoke, and the nicotine is absorbed into the lungs.

The electronic cigarette, or e-cigarette, is sold with cartridges of nicotine and flavorings. Several brands and varieties of the e-cigarette are now sold in the United States. Here, the e-cigarette is usually sold as a way to get nicotine in places where smoking is not allowed, although some may sell it as a way to quit smoking. The cartridges are sold in different doses of nicotine, from high doses to no nicotine at all.

There are no published clinical trials that suggest the e-cigarette might work as a way to help smokers quit. No clinical trials have been submitted to the FDA. As of early 2009, the FDA had not ruled as to whether e-cigarettes are medical devices, but it is investigating. There may also be questions about how safe it is to inhale some of the flavorings and other substances in the nicotine mists. Even substances that are safe to eat can harm delicate tissues inside the lungs.

Like other forms of nicotine, e-cigarettes and nicotine cartridges can be toxic to children or pets. They can also pose a choking hazard.

Nicotine Water and Nicotine Wafers

These products are advertised as ways to get nicotine in places where smoking is not allowed. They are not marketed as aids to quitting smoking, but questions about their safety have been raised. Some of these formulas can be quite dangerous if accidentally taken by children or pets, so they must be stored carefully.

Support Keeps You Going Strong

If you're serious about quitting, medication alone isn't enough. Tobacco users who try to quit without support usually have a harder time. Research shows that adding social support to medication treatment can boost your long-term quitting success. Including either individual or group counseling in your quitting plan is much more effective than no counseling.

With so many quitting support options, it's critical to enlist the support of your doctor and other resources in finding a program or group that suits your needs.

▶ GET ORGANIZED

Organized support can help you—

- learn to predict and avoid temptation.
- create strategies for handling bad moods.
- make lifestyle changes to reduce stress and improve your quality of life.
- use mental and physical activities to cope with smoking urges.
- hear others' experiences with and tips for handling stresses, triggers, and cravings.

▶ THE LOWDOWN ON STOP-SMOKING MEDICATIONS

Type of Medication	Prescription Needed?	Dosage
NICOTINE PATCH (transdermal nicotine system)	NO	15–22 mg/day for 4 weeks; may taper to 5–14 mg/day for 4 weeks. Use for 2–5 months. Available as a 16-hour patch or 24-hour patch.
NICOTINE GUM (nicotine polacrilex)	NO	2 or 4 mg. Use as needed, or use 1–2 pieces an hour on a fixed schedule, no more than 20 pieces/day. Taper the dose before stopping use. Use for 1–3 months (no more than 6 months).
NICOTINE NASAL SPRAY	YES	1–2 doses an hour (one spray into each nostril is a dose). Use for 3 months; gradually taper off (use for a maximum of 6 months).
NICOTINE INHALER	YES	6–16 cartridges/day for 3 months, then taper off for 3 months (use for a maximum of 6 months). One cartridge delivers the amount of nicotine found in 2 cigarettes.
ZYBAN (bupropion hydrochloride)	YES	Begin taking 1–2 weeks before quitting; after quitting, continue for 7–12 weeks or longer.
CHANTIX (varenicline)	YES	One 0.5 mg/day for the first 3 days, then twice a day for the next 4 days. Starting the second week, 1 mg each morning and evening. The drug is usually given for 12 weeks; another 12 weeks may be required.

How to Use	Why to Use	Disadvantages
Apply to skin every day. A constant dose of nicotine is absorbed through the skin.	Easy to use. Few side effects.	Releases nicotine more slowly than other options. Can cause skin irritation; 24-hour patch may cause sleep disturbance.
Chew slowly, then "park" in the cheek. Nicotine is absorbed through the mouth lining.	Convenient. Can use as needed. Nicotine is absorbed within minutes.	Can't eat or drink (except for water) just before, during, or after use. Talk with your dentist if you have sensitive dental work or jaw problems.
Spray into nose.	Quick nicotine delivery controls sudden cravings.	Nasal and sinus irritation are common. Not for people with allergies, sinus conditions, or asthma.
Puff on inhaler.	Few side effects. Delivers nicotine as quickly as gum. Can satisfy hand-to-mouth urges.	May cause coughing or mouth or throat irritation. Not for people with asthma or diseases that cause airway spasms.
Take 1 pill in the morning, 1 in the late afternoon.	Easy to use. Few side effects. May be more helpful when used with other nicotine replacement therapy.	May cause dry mouth or sleep disturbance. Do not use if you have seizures/eating disorders, if you are taking Wellbutrin, MAO inhibitors, or other medications that contain bupropion, or if you are pregnant or breastfeeding.
Take pills according to dosage regimen.	Easy to use. May double the chance of quitting.	May cause headaches, nausea, vomiting, trouble sleeping, unusual dreams, flatulence, changes in taste, thoughts of suicide, depressed mood. Tell your doctor about emotional changes such as depression, agitation, or thoughts of suicide.

Strength in Numbers

When other people know about your commitment you may be more likely to stick to it and stay focused on your goal.

Stop-smoking programs help smokers recognize and cope with problems that come up during quitting and provide support and encouragement in staying quit. In general, more intense programs have the highest success rates, so look for a program that has the following:

- session length: at least 20 to 30 minutes
- session frequency: at least 4 to 7 sessions
- session duration: at least 2 weeks

▶ BE AWARE

Not all stop-smoking programs are ethical. Be careful of programs that do any of the following:

- Promise instant, easy success with no effort on your part
- Use injections or pills, especially "secret" ingredients
- Charge a very high fee — check with the Better Business Bureau if you have doubts
- Are not willing to provide references from people who have taken the class

---

Finding Support Groups. Many stop-smoking support groups are free. Others charge a fee. To find stop-smoking groups in your area, try one or more of the following options:

- Call any of the national groups (or their local offices) in the Resource Guide beginning on page 111.

- Call your local hospitals to find out about stop-smoking groups in your area.

- Look up "Smokers Information and Treatment Centers" in the yellow pages of the phone book.

- Call the American Cancer Society at 800-227-2345 for local resources.

The Internet has brought millions of people a new world of communication, including some very helpful stop-smoking chat groups and sites. But beware of any group or literature on the Internet that "guarantees" you'll stop smoking.

■ **in the community:** Some communities have a Nicotine Anonymous group that holds regular meetings. (See the Web site: nicotine-anonymous.org.) This group applies the principles of Alcoholics Anonymous to the addiction of smoking. There is no fee to participate.

The American Cancer Society (800-227-2345; cancer.org), the American Lung Association (lungusa.org), or your local Health Department often sponsors stop-smoking classes.

A variety of other health-serving organizations and community- and hospital-based groups offer information on how to quit and where to go for help. Support groups are available to provide emotional support, friendship, and understanding.

■ **at work:** Call the human resources office where you work; your company may offer information about stop-smoking programs. The American Cancer Society's Great American Smokeout® is held in many companies each November. If your company has an Employee Assistance Program, its counselors can direct you to community stop-smoking programs. Your employer might pay for you to attend a program or reimburse you for the cost of the program.

Call for Help: Telephone Counseling

Through telephone counseling, you can talk to a counselor one-on-one about quitting smoking. Telephone counseling services, or quitlines, are often sponsored by state health departments. A counselor can support you, give you information, answer questions, and even help you come up with a plan that will work for you. Many counselors have backgrounds in counseling and have gone through a training program. Some are ex-smokers.

Quitlines give callers a place to start and the support to move forward each step of the way. A helpful quitline offers callers the following services:

- someone to turn to so you don't have to quit alone
- a sense of privacy through telephone-based counseling
- one-on-one motivational support throughout the quitting process
- up-to-date smoking cessation information
- free access anytime, day or night
- referrals to local support resources

The American Cancer Society offers telephone services for tobacco users interested in quitting. Contact the Society at 800-227-2345 (cancer.org) for more information.

Your Quitting Plan

You may choose to use one or a combination of methods to quit smoking, including self-help classes or counseling, group sessions, nicotine replacement therapy, or other medications.

Think through the most crucial parts of your quitting plan and commit to trying them by writing them down here:

- Will you quit cold turkey, or have you opted to taper down?

  _____

- If you will use a stop-smoking medication, which one will you use?

  _____

  _____

- Will you use any other methods to support your quit attempt?

  _____

  _____

- Will you rely on some type of organized support? What type?

  _____

  _____

CHAPTER 3

Countdown to Quitting

J UST BY DECIDING TO STOP SMOKING, you've taken your first step along the path to a smoke-free life. Most people who relapse start smoking within the first week after quitting, when withdrawal symptoms are strongest and their bodies are still dependent on nicotine. Planning carefully will help you through your first big challenge: the beginning of your quit attempt.

Change Your Mind About Smoking

One of the toughest parts of getting ready to quit is changing your mindset about smoking. After your Quit Day, you'll consider smoking to be absolutely off limits.

Feeling afraid, sad, or angry about quitting is normal. Try to keep in mind your many specific reasons for quitting. Stay strong. Many people who went into their Quit Days with mixed feelings or doubts became nonsmokers. A positive, no-excuses attitude can help you succeed in quitting.

Cope Without a Smoke

You work through challenges every day. When you quit smoking, you'll simply work through daily challenges without smoking. You can help avoid being tempted to smoke when you come across common stresses by getting ready to face them.

Get Ready for Cravings

As soon as you stop using tobacco, nicotine and other tobacco poisons start to leave your body. If you're hooked on nicotine, your body will send your brain a message—through withdrawal symptoms—saying, "Hello, I need nicotine!" In this chapter and the next we'll talk about how to be prepared for some strong cravings so you won't slip up.

The Smokers Around You

You'll be working hard to keep from smoking again, but some of your friends, family, or coworkers may still smoke. The smokers in your life may be worried you'll judge them for smoking or pester them to stop, too. They may wonder how your kicking the habit will affect your time together. They may not be glad you're quitting or may feel uncomfortable helping you quit. And you may not feel right about turning to them for support when you feel tempted to smoke.

For the first few weeks of your quit attempt, you may be especially vulnerable to smoking again. Avoid places where others are smoking if you can. Tell yourself it's okay to leave if people start smoking.

The Picture of Health

It's normal to gain a few pounds as nicotine leaves your body. But not everyone gains weight when they quit, and people who do usually gain only five or ten pounds. Some medications that can help you quit smoking may also help prevent those unwanted pounds.

> ### ▶ WHY DO PEOPLE GAIN WEIGHT WHEN THEY QUIT SMOKING?
>
> • Nicotine suppresses your appetite.
>
> • Nicotine speeds up the system and makes people burn calories more quickly.
>
> • People often snack more when they quit because they feel bored, angry, lonely, or stressed.
>
> • A smoker is often used to having a cigarette in his or her mouth and may use food as a substitute when quitting.

A small amount of weight gain is really a matter of perspective. It's much worse for your health to continue smoking than it is to gain a few pounds. Smoking causes more than 400,000 deaths each year in the United States.

Eat and Run. You know that quitting smoking is the best thing that you can do for yourself and those around you. While you're quitting, it may be easier to focus on ways to stay healthy than to worry about your weight. These steps will help you condition your body before and during the quitting process:

- Start a modest, regular exercise program.

- Drink plenty of fluids.

- Eat fruits and vegetables.

- Limit fat intake.

- Get enough sleep.

Gradually improving your eating habits may be easier than making many changes at once. Changing your eating habits too quickly can add to the stress of quitting smoking.

Sticking to an eating schedule can help you keep extra weight off, since skipping meals and becoming very hungry before eating might cause you to overeat. To keep yourself healthy, eat a variety of low-fat foods and low-calorie snacks instead of high-calorie, high-fat treats. In Chapter 4, you'll read a few other simple tactics for avoiding weight gain.

Hand-to-Mouth. If you feel hungry between meals, drink water or low-calorie drinks or eat sugarless candy and fruit. Before your Quit Day, consider cutting back on coffee, caffeinated and sugary sodas, and alcohol, all of which can make you want to light up. Also think about buying or making these types of low-calorie foods for snacking:

- sticks of carrots or celery
- lemon or lime water
- coffee-flavored candy
- sugarless gum
- low-fat cottage cheese
- fruity or herbal teas

- strong mints
- apple slices
- raisins
- rice cakes
- orange sections
- pretzels

- sunflower seeds
- licorice
- air-popped popcorn
- lemon drops
- butterscotch candies
- lollipops
- ice
- mini candy canes
- flavored decaffeinated coffee

Get Physical. To keep fit as you quit, hit the road, the trail, or the gym for some exercise. Try activities like walking, dancing, skating, basketball, biking, hiking, swimming, running, weightlifting, or exercise classes like aerobics, yoga, spinning, kickboxing, or sculpting. Keeping active for 30 minutes a day 3 to 4 times a week will help you get more fit while also remaining smoke-free.

Exercise also helps cut down on stress, which sends many people back to cigarettes again. It can also help you get rid of the temporary blues that some smokers experience when they quit.

You might be able to pump up your motivation for exercising by getting active *before* your Quit Day. That

▶ WHAT'S THE PLAN OF ATTACK?

It's a good idea not only to plan what you'll do when a craving hits, but also to practice your strategy before you quit. On your Quit Day, having to spend a long time searching for a substitute for smoking is a recipe for disaster. Have snacks, drinks, and things to fidget with on hand, and keep a list handy of ways to deal with urges.

way you'll feel better sooner, and when you quit you'll already be well on your way to being more fit. If you don't already exercise regularly, check with your doctor before starting an exercise program.

Get a Handle on Stress

Smokers who try to quit but smoke again often mention stress as one of the reasons they end up going back to smoking. Whether at work, at home, or on the road between the two, everyone—smokers and non-smokers—experiences some pressure or anxiety. Many smokers use nicotine to help them cope.

You can help your body and mind get used to relaxing before Quit Day. Check your local newspaper, library, or bookstore for stress-management classes or self-help books. Plan specific ways to handle stress. Think of things you can do instead of smoking when stress hits, such as one of the following activities:

- chew gum
- squeeze a rubber ball
- take a hot shower or bath
- take a five-minute walk
- read a book
- talk it through

Take a Break. You deserve to take time out of your day specifically to relax. Find a few moments to calm your mind and consciously give yourself a break from daily pressures. Find a distraction or call a friend or someone in your support group to talk through any challenges or stress.

Breathe Deeply and Relax. Deep breathing exercises can help you get through a stressful moment without lighting up. Deep abdominal breathing involves breathing from the lower part of the abdomen. Slow rhythmic breathing involves staring at an object or closing your eyes and concentrating on breathing or on a peaceful scene.

If you find yourself in a stressful situation, step away, then take a slow, deep breath for five seconds, hold it in as you count to five, then let it out slowly for five seconds. Doing this for a few minutes can help you slow down and calm down.

Quiet Your Mind. Spiritual practices like prayer and meditation are often helpful parts of drug and alcohol addiction programs and are integral to 12-step recovery programs. These spiritual principles can be applied to quitting smoking and can help with stress reduction.

Meditation is a way of relaxing the body and calming the mind to create a sense of well-being. A person meditates by concentrating on a pleasant idea or thought, chanting a phrase or special sound (sometimes called a mantra), or focusing on the sound of his or her own breathing. There are many variations, and a person can meditate alone or with an instructor, yoga master, doctor, or mental health professional. Some clinics at major medical centers and local hospitals offer meditation as a form of behavioral medicine.

Get Ready for Quit Day

From now until your Quit Day, consider spending about 30 minutes a day getting your mind, body, home, work, and support group preparations ready. Focusing and preparing your surroundings and yourself will maximize your chances of quitting.

Drum Up Support

Support can make a big difference as you quit smoking. Informal support from those around you can really help you stay strong.

Set Other People Straight. Tell your family, friends, and coworkers that you're going to quit and ask for their support while you're quitting and after you quit. Explain what a challenge quitting may be and how much help they can be to you.

Tell those around you about your plan to quit. Ask them to help you stay away from cigarettes and to support you in specific ways:

- Please don't smoke in the house.
- Please don't keep cigarettes in the house.
- Please don't smoke in the car.
- Please don't smoke around me.
- Please don't offer me cigarettes.
- Please say no if I ask for a cigarette.

To thank them for their help, you might make a special dinner or treat them to a movie.

Look to former smokers for support, too. They've been through what you're going through and can support you in unique ways when you have a hard time not smoking.

You might want to ask one family member, one coworker, and one friend to serve as your core support group. Ask them to help support you in specific ways.

▶ WHEN I NEED HELP

Ask a few close friends if you can turn to them to talk you out of going back to tobacco. Write down what you think will keep you from smoking and let these people know what support you need.

EXAMPLE:

Name _____ *David* _____

The type of help I'd like from you is ___ *Remind me that*
I want to travel with the money I spend on cigarettes
each year (over $1000). Tell me I can get through this
challenge without smoking! _____

Name

The type of help I'd like from you is

_____

_____

_____

Name

The type of help I'd like from you is

_____

_____

_____

Name

The type of help I'd like from you is

_____

_____

_____

Your Danger Zone

Simple daily events like finishing a meal, talking on the phone, driving, or talking with friends can often trigger your urge to smoke. Recognizing your smoking triggers will help you resist them.

Steer Clear of Triggers. You learned *why* you reach for a cigarette by taking the "Why Test" in Chapter 1. Now think about *when* and *where* you're most vulnerable to smoking. You may want to develop a list of certain people and places that tempt you to smoke and that you could avoid, especially during the first few days.

Resist Temptation. While you quit, you can avoid certain situations when you'll want to smoke. But eventually you'll need to face these situations again, so you'll want to know how to get through your triggers without smoking.

An important part of resisting triggers is separating the smoking habit from your daily routine. You can practice doing this before your Quit Day by putting off smoking a habitual cigarette—the habit of smoking a cigarette when you're in a certain place, at a certain time, or when you're with a certain someone.

> ▶ **TRIAL RUN**
>
> Even if you're going to quit cold turkey, you might want to try to resist the urge to smoke before you officially quit — at first for an hour, then for a morning or an evening, and then for 24 hours. That way, before you quit smoking altogether you can figure out how to best deal with the urge to smoke.

▶ BREAK THE LINK

Part of facing your triggers is breaking the link between the trigger and your smoking. Think about the times and places you usually smoke. What could you do instead of smoking when you find yourself in a "danger zone?"

If you usually smoke . . .

After lunch
(Plan to eat lunch at local delis and nonsmoking restaurants, or at your desk?)

In the car
(Plan to take public transportation or vary your route to work so you're more conscious that you're making a change?)

With coworkers
(Plan to take a short walk with a nonsmoking coworker instead?)

When drinking alcohol
(Drink a lot of water and other nonalcoholic drinks? Avoiding alcohol for the first few months after quitting will help you quit.)

When . . .

_____
_____
_____
_____

What can you do instead?

_____
_____
_____

_____
_____
_____
_____
_____

_____
_____
_____

_____
_____
_____
_____
_____

_____
_____
_____
_____

Instead of smoking when you get off work like you usually do, for instance, tell yourself you won't light up the "after work" cigarette until after you get home. The craving will likely have passed by then. Try taking smoking out of the picture when you feel like lighting up a habitual smoke. See the "Break the Link" section on page 71 for more ideas.

Mix It Up a Little. Changing your routine when you first quit can help you stick to a nonsmoking agenda. Rather than smoking when you wake up in the morning, try drinking hot tea or eating breakfast, jumping in the shower first thing, washing your face with cold water, or otherwise shaking up your morning habits a little.

If you usually smoke with your morning coffee, make a point of drinking your coffee in a different place than you did when you smoked. You might drink your coffee standing up, in a different room, or while looking out the window, for example.

Stay Busy: Nonsmoking Activities

Many of the ways you might cope with stress (calling a friend), urges (distraction), or weight gain (exercise) can also help you keep busy and keep your mind off cigarettes.

When you go to a smoke-free place like a movie theater, museum, library, mall or store, or religious service, you won't be able to smoke. You can also stay busy by exercising, walking the dog, playing ball, spending time with other nonsmokers, playing video games, or calling a friend.

Plan Rewards for Yourself

You deserve to be good to yourself as you quit. Plan to do something fun every day as a reward for not smoking. Whether it's going somewhere, seeing someone, taking time for yourself, or buying something, write each reward on your calendar and treat each reward as an important appointment.

If you're used to rewarding yourself with a cigarette, plan new ways to reward yourself.

- Go fishing.
- Play a new computer game.
- Visit a friend.
- See a new movie or art exhibit.
- Listen to a new CD.
- Take a hot bath or shower and relax.
- Read outside.
- Buy something you've always wanted.
- _____
- _____
- _____
- _____
- _____
- _____

Choose something you really want to do on your Quit Day and write it on your calendar. Plan to go to lunch with nonsmoking friends to celebrate, schedule a dinner date after work, or go on a hike. Keep yourself busy so you aren't thinking about smoking.

The Day Before Quit Day

You're almost ready for your Quit Day. You've worked through many of the challenges you might face as you quit. How else can you make the first few days a little easier on yourself?

- Wash your clothes and bedding to get rid of the stale smell of cigarettes, which can linger a long time.

- Do any errands or chores now so you won't have to deal with them later, like paying bills, catching up on a work project, or finishing a chore at home.

- Get a good night's sleep each night this first week so you're well rested.

Reducing a few everyday stresses will help you manage the challenge of quitting.

Think About Tomorrow. Think through the kind of day you'll have tomorrow. Where will you be? What will you be doing? Who will you be with? Imagine what you'll do at every step during the day. What times and situations might make you want to smoke?

It might help to reread your "Break the Link" worksheet on page 71. Practice what you'll say or do when you are tempted or stressed. Think through simple ways to cope with each situation without smoking.

Get Motivated. Look over "My Quitting Reminders" on pages 20–21 and pause to think about each of your reasons for quitting. Don't forget to post your lists where you expect to need motivation.

Put Out Your Last Cigarette. Before you go to bed, smoke one last cigarette if you need to. Throw away tobacco, lighters, matches, and ashtrays. Make sure you've searched your house, office, car, coat pockets, and purse for stashes. Now get a good night's sleep so you'll be ready for your first day as a nonsmoker.

> ▶ **GET READY**
>
> Are you and your environment ready for your Quit Day? This checklist will help you review the practical coping ideas in this chapter.
>
> **Your *Bag of Tricks:***
>
> What will you put in your *Bag of Tricks*?
>
> ❏ Nicotine gum, nasal spray, the patch, lozenges, or inhaler
>
> ❏ Support group numbers (800-227-2345, numbers for members of your personal support group, and/or others)
>
> ❏ An encouraging note from a friend or from your child
>
> ❏ "My Quitting Reminders" on pages 20–21
>
> ❏ "When I Need Help" on page 69
>
> ❏ "Break the Link" on page 71
>
> ❏ _____
>
> ❏ _____
>
> *(continued)*

Cravings:

❏ Are you ready to distract yourself from cravings by keeping busy with other activities like walking, playing on the computer, or talking to a friend?

❏ Do you have gum, hard candies, toothpicks, and low-calorie drinks on hand to chew, bite on, or drink instead of smoking?

❏ Do you have a headache reliever, throat lozenges, and cough drops handy in case you feel withdrawal symptoms?

❏ Are you ready to delay for 10 minutes whenever you feel a craving?

Support:

❏ Do you have stop-smoking medications ready to go?

❏ If you are using bupropion (Zyban) or varenicline (Chantix), have you been taking it as directed?

❏ Have you joined an organized support group or set up other counseling services (like Quitline support)?

❏ Have you explained what you need to your personal support group members?

❏ Have you asked the smokers in your life not to smoke around you and not to give you cigarettes?

Exercise:

❏ Do you have exercise clothes and shoes ready to go?

(continued)

❑ Have you booked an appointment with yourself each day to exercise?

❑ Do you have exercise videos or hand weights available?

❑ Do you know the local exercise class schedule?

❑ Do you know the community swimming pool's hours?

Nonsmoking Surroundings:

❑ Do you have a movie schedule handy?

❑ Do you know the hours your local museum is open?

❑ If you're interested in religious services, do you know where and when they take place?

❑ Do you have any errands to do at local shops or the mall?

❑ Do you have meals scheduled at nonsmoking restaurants?

Rewards:

❑ Do you have music to listen to that makes you happy or relaxed?

❑ Have you listed a few things to buy for yourself?

❑ Have you found any nonsmoking pool halls?

❑ Do you have any new places you'd like to go?

❑ If you'll reward yourself with a massage, have you scheduled it?

❑ Do you have a schedule for your favorite sports team's games?

Quit Day

It's Quit Day! Today you become a nonsmoker. You may spend most of your time and energy simply *not smoking* today. That's okay. Just hold on through this first day. Each day of not smoking will become easier.

Put Your Plans into Action

Today's the day to follow through with the plans you laid out in Chapter 3. Here's a step-by-step review:

- **Cope with smoking triggers.** If you can't avoid your triggers, rely on the tactics and ideas in the "If You Used to Smoke When . . ." worksheet on pages 82–84 in this chapter.

- **Relieve stress.** Take a break, breathe deeply, and try meditating or relaxing. Make a special effort to get plenty of rest for the next couple of weeks.

- **Rely on support.** Rely on the support network you set up in Chapter 3. Go to your "When I Need Help" contact sheet on page 69 whenever you need help working through a craving.

- **Find alternatives to smoking.** Occupy your hands by playing with a pencil or a marble. Use oral substitutions like cinnamon sticks, celery or carrots, or hard candy if you miss the feeling of having something in your mouth.

- **Keep busy.** Hobbies that keep your hands busy and require concentration can help distract you from the urge to smoke. Needlework, woodworking, playing the piano, working a puzzle, playing a video game, or surfing the Internet can also help keep your mind off smoking.

▶ QUICK FIXES FOR EVERYDAY CHALLENGES

Relieve Stress

You may need some quick fixes for coping with stress. When you find yourself upset, angry, or anxious and wanting a cigarette, try one or all of the following:

- Take 10 deep breaths.
- Take a hot shower or bath.
- Walk, skate, or bike around the block and breathe in the fresh air.
- Work in the yard or your home.
- Light incense or a candle instead of a cigarette.
- Shoot hoops.
- Stretch fully, bend your spine, and roll your head gently in circles.
- Work out with a punching bag.
- Visualize a soothing situation and let your body go limp.
- Think about consciously slowing down your thoughts and actions and relaxing your body.

(continued)

Start Moving

Walking and jogging are easy ways to add activity to your day. And you can do them almost anywhere:

- Get off the bus one stop before you usually do and walk.
- Walk or jog with a friend during lunch.
- Run or walk while exercising the dog.
- Walk or jog while pushing your child in a stroller.

Eat Smart

The following "tricks" can help you avoid gaining weight and distract you from smoking:

- Drink a glass of water before eating a meal.
- Reduce your portions.
- Get up from the table as soon as you're finished eating.
- Brush your teeth or use mouthwash immediately after a meal.
- Avoid sugary and fatty foods, which can make you want to smoke.

- **Get physical.** Simple ways to become more physically active include gardening, house repairs, mowing the lawn, playing with the kids, cleaning, and taking the stairs instead of the elevator.

- **Eat smart.** Eating small meals throughout the day maintains constant blood sugar levels and helps prevent you from feeling the urge to smoke. Avoid sugary foods, spicy foods, and alcohol. These can trigger a desire for cigarettes.

▶ IF YOU USED TO SMOKE WHEN . . .

Consider the following tactics for getting through triggers without smoking. Feel free to write in any other ideas you have.

If you used to smoke when you talked on the phone, try the following tactics:

- Tell yourself "I don't smoke" before picking up the phone.
- Keep a list of the reasons for quitting by the phone and review it.
- Stand if you usually sit while you talk; sit if you usually stand.
- Walk around or straighten the house while you talk.
- Doodle on a scratch pad.
- File your nails.
- Whittle on a piece of wood.
- Fold a sheet of paper into a tiny square, unfold, and repeat.
- Tear a sheet of paper slowly and carefully into tiny pieces.

- _____
- _____
- _____

If you used to smoke at the computer, try the following tactics:

- Create a screen saver that says "I'm a nonsmoker."
- Bookmark a stop-smoking Web site or bulletin board and visit it often.

(continued)

- If cigarettes helped you concentrate, keep a paperweight or other object next to the keyboard and focus on it.

- _____

If you used to smoke during work breaks, try the following tactics:

- Take your break, but spend it with a nonsmoking friend in a nonsmoking spot.
- Read a newspaper or magazine during your break.
- Sit quietly with your eyes closed and take an imaginary mini-vacation.
- If you do spend time with smokers, bring your "Bag of Tricks" from page 75.

- _____
- _____

If you used to smoke when you socialized, try the following tactics:

- Sit next to nonsmokers in the group.
- If you usually drink alcohol, drink nonalcoholic drinks at least half the time.
- Get up and walk around often.
- Take deep breaths.
- Chew on a straw or toothpick.

- _____
- _____

If you used to smoke in the car, try the following tactics:

- Take the ashtray and lighter out of the car.

(continued)

- Sing along with your favorite songs.
- Roll down the windows and breathe fresh air.
- Listen to a book on tape.
- _____
- _____

Create a Smoke-Free Environment

As you prepared to quit smoking, you got rid of smoking reminders like ashtrays, cigarette stashes, and the smell of stale smoke. Now that it's your Quit Day, you can develop an even cleaner, fresher nonsmoking environment at work and at home.

Ask family members and friends not to smoke in your house or car. Have gum or mints available as an alternative to lighting up. If family members or visitors feel they absolutely must smoke, ask them to smoke outside.

Get Over Smoking

Any withdrawal symptoms you feel are really symptoms of the recovery process. If your body is craving nicotine, it means it's healing.

Most relapses take place the first week after quitting, when withdrawal symptoms are strongest and the body is still dependent on nicotine. Equipping yourself with all the available resources will help you get through this difficult time. Withdrawal symptoms and the urge to smoke will pass whether you smoke or not.

Your Body Is Adjusting

Your body goes through a lot of changes as it gets rid of all the tobacco ingredients it has grown to love. It only makes sense that it's bitter about being deprived, and that it sends you angry messages. That's what withdrawal symptoms are.

If they occur, withdrawal symptoms usually start within a few hours of the last cigarette and peak about 48 to 72 hours later. They can last for a few days to several weeks. After that, your body will begin to forget about nicotine and you'll feel better. Very few people have every withdrawal symptom, and no one ever experiences all of them at once.

You may not have any of these experiences, but if you do, don't worry. It's normal. As your body adjusts to the absence of nicotine, you may experience some combination of these symptoms:

- **Headache:** Your body is adjusting to increased oxygen in your system and less carbon monoxide.

- **Dizziness or lightheadedness:** Your body is receiving more oxygen than it's used to.

- **Constipation:** The intestines will adjust to a lack of nicotine after a short period.

- **Difficulty concentrating:** Your brain takes time to adapt to working without being stimulated by nicotine.

- **Irritability:** Nicotine affects the chemistry of the brain and central nervous system, so it can affect your mood. At first you may feel nervous or touchy. Try exercising—it may help you feel better.

- **Tiredness:** Nicotine is a stimulant, so when you aren't smoking anymore, you may feel tired.

- **Inability to sleep soundly:** Nicotine affects brain wave function, so you may wake up during the night. You may also dream about smoking.

- **Hunger:** You may think the urge you feel to smoke is really a hunger pang.

- **Coughing:** Coughing helps the body get rid of the mucus clogging your lungs.

- **Dry mouth:** When you stop smoking, your body won't produce as much mucus, so your mouth may feel dry.

- **Depression:** Some ex-smokers say that giving up cigarettes is like losing a best friend. Bouts of crying are common. But these sad feelings will pass. Smoking isn't the solution.

You may not feel exactly the same as others do who are quitting. Any of these feelings you have will go away, so hang in there. Give yourself a chance to get over smoking.

Your Mind May Play Tricks on You

Like a mischievous devil on your shoulder, your mind may come up with rationalizations for smoking—thoughts that seem to make sense at the time but aren't based on facts. If you feel yourself finding reasons why it's okay to smoke, knock that devil off your shoulder. You're a nonsmoker now, and smoking cigarettes is not an option.

▶ MIND GAMES

If you allow yourself to rationalize or make excuses for smoking even one cigarette on or after your Quit Day, you're likely to become a regular smoker again. Expect the rationalizations below when you feel withdrawal symptoms. That way you'll be ready and able to see through them.

Typical physical withdrawal symptoms

- Depression
- Frustration
- Irritability and anger
- Trouble sleeping
- Difficulty concentrating
- Restlessness
- Headache
- Tiredness
- Increased appetite

Typical psychological rationalizations

- I'll just have one to get through this rough spot.
- Today is not a good day; I'll quit tomorrow.
- It's my only vice.
- How bad is smoking really?
- Uncle Harry smoked all his life, and he lived to be over 90.
- Air pollution is probably just as bad.
- You've got to die of *something*.
- Life is no fun without smoking.
- I'll gain weight if I stop.

As you go through your first few days without smoking, write down any rationalizations as they come up and recognize them for what they are: messages that can trap you into going back to smoking.

Talk to yourself. If you have the urge to smoke, tell yourself "no." Say it out loud. Practice doing this a few times, and listen to yourself. Here are some other pep talks you may want to rely on today and in the days to come to talk yourself out of smoking:

- "I will not smoke today."
- "Other people have quit, and I can, too."
- "Smoking is not an option."
- "This craving will pass in a few minutes whether I smoke or not."
- "I am a nonsmoker."
- "I'm too strong to be tied down by smoking."
- "One cigarette does matter."
- "I don't want to let down my friends and family."
- "I'm too tough to give in to a craving."
- "I want to live a long life."

Withdrawal Relief. Time, home remedies, and stop-smoking medicines like those outlined in Chapter 2 can all make withdrawal easier. Many people use a combination of these to work through symptoms. Personal care and over-the-counter remedies can also help ease withdrawal pangs.

Pump Up Your Motivation

Remind yourself why you started thinking about quitting, and don't think of giving up cigarettes forever. Just concentrate on one day at a time. Tell yourself, "I won't smoke today."

▶ TO THE RESCUE

Here are some of the most common withdrawal symptoms and ways you might handle them. Feel free to add your own ideas of ways to cope with specific withdrawal symptoms.

Headache	• Take Tylenol or your usual headache reliever.
	• Use relaxation techniques.
Dizziness or lightheadedness	• Close your eyes for a moment and breathe slowly.
	• Sit down and rest for a minute.
	• _____
	• _____
Sore throat	• Suck on lozenges or hard candies.
	• Drink plenty of liquids.
	• _____
	• _____
Cough	• Use cough drops.
	• Drink plenty of liquids.
	• _____
	• _____
Trouble sleeping	• Cut down on caffeine.
	• Read a dull book.
	• _____
	• _____

(continued)

Depression	• Talk to a friend.
	• Rely on your support group.
	• _____
	• _____
Constipation	• Increase fruit, fiber, and fluid intake.
	• Exercise.
	• _____
	• _____
Feeling nervous or irritable	• Cut down on caffeine.
	• Breathe deeply.
	• Take warm showers or baths.
	• Use a punching bag.
	• _____
	• _____
Difficulty concentrating	• Make a "to do" list.
	• Take extra time to get things done.
	• _____
	• _____

Your Personal Reasons for Quitting

You've posted your "My Quitting Reminders" list from pages 20–21 where you can see it, and you've tucked a copy into your wallet. When you feel vulnerable to smoking again, rely on this list as a reminder of your reasons for quitting. These reasons are the root of your motivation for quitting.

▶ WHAT YOU CAN DO INSTEAD OF SMOKING: A CHEAT SHEET

Use this at-a-glance list to remind yourself of the many ways you can get through the challenges of quitting smoking with success.

Prevent weight gain:
- Brush your teeth after eating.
- Drink cold water.

Manage your mouth:
- Chew gum.
- Eat hard candy.
- Chew on a straw or toothpick.

Keep hands busy:
- Straighten a paper clip.
- Fidget with a straw.
- Play with a small toy.

Cope:
- Take a deep breath.
- Go for a walk or run.
- Scream in the shower or in the car.
- Punch a pillow.
- Talk to a friend.

Distract:
- Take a drive.
- Go to a movie.
- Sleep or take a short nap.

Avoid:
- Leave a tempting situation.
- Spend time in nonsmoking spots.
- Don't drink alcohol or coffee.

Relax:
- Write to a friend.
- Take a walk.
- Take a bath.
- Watch TV.

Refresh:
- Read.
- Wash your face.
- Exercise.

Encourage:
- Remind yourself: "I can do this."
- Remember cravings will pass.
- Remember why you want to quit.

▶ DAILY CHECKLIST

Make copies of this checklist and use them to keep on track every day. And stay alert: People sometimes get cocky and forget about the tips and tricks they've learned. Check off each item each day to remind yourself of the steps that make quitting possible.
Date:

I'll deal with withdrawal:

❏ Nicotine patch — I'm wearing it.

❏ Nicotine gum, nasal spray, lozenge, or inhaler — I have it handy.

❏ Bupropion (Zyban) or varenicline (Chantix) — I have taken it today.

❏ Home remedies — I have them handy.

I'll make new routines:

❏ I know what I am going to do in situations when I used to smoke.

❏ Alternatives — I have distractions nearby to keep my hands and mouth busy.

❏ Activities — I'll keep moving and improve my health while not smoking.

I'll watch out for tempting situations:

❏ Avoid them — I'll get away from the situation as gracefully as possible.

❏ Alter them — I'll change what I would normally do until the feeling goes away.

(continued)

American Cancer Society

❏ Decline offers for cigarettes—I'm a nonsmoker now.

In general, I'll do the following things:

❏ Rely on my support system.

❏ Turn negative thoughts around so they don't bring me down.

❏ Spend more time with people who don't smoke.

❏ Go easy on myself because this is a big change.

❏ Remind myself of my personal reasons for quitting.

At the end of the day, I'll ask myself the following questions:

❏ What went well? I'll do those things again tomorrow.

❏ What needs to improve? I can change it.

❏ What will my day be like tomorrow? I'll be ready for it.

First thing tomorrow, I'll use this checklist again.

The Immediate Benefits of Quitting

Within 12 hours after you have your last cigarette, your body will begin to heal itself. The levels of carbon monoxide and nicotine in your system decrease, and your heart and lungs begin to repair the damage caused by cigarette smoke. Just think: those positive changes are happening in your body right now simply because you're not smoking.

Treat Yourself

It's the end of your Quit Day. Way to go! You've made it a full day without smoking. On page 73, you planned out rewards for yourself. What's the reward you have planned for today? As you enjoy the reward you chose, think to yourself, "I'm really proud of myself for quitting. I deserve this. I'm working hard at being a nonsmoker." Talking to yourself like this may sound silly, but being proud of your hard work isn't. Don't forget to take a minute to think about all you're accomplishing.

CHAPTER 5

Your Smoke-Free Life

BY NOW YOU PROBABLY KNOW that deciding to quit smoking and staying quit are different things. Not smoking isn't always easy. But it is always good for you and will help you live a longer, healthier life. That's why it can help to stay on top of the things that might threaten to get you smoking again.

Your life as a nonsmoker will get easier, as long as you do the following:

- Stay aware of tempting situations.
- Remember to practice the quitting skills you've learned so far.
- Think of yourself as a nonsmoker.

This chapter builds on what you know about coping with challenges and can help you build a healthy and smoke-free lifestyle.

The Habit of Not Smoking

Like any other habit, it takes time for not smoking to become a part of your routine. But unlike most other habits, not smoking also takes some conscious effort and practice.

Remember Your Coping Skills

These are the major coping skills you've learned to use as you fight the urge to smoke. Use at least one when you're tempted by nicotine.

1. **Never forget why you quit smoking.** Go back to your list of reasons for quitting. Look at this list frequently—especially when you feel the urge to smoke. Your personal reasons for quitting are also the best reasons to stay a nonsmoker.

2. **Know when you're rationalizing.** We tend to remember the good parts of smoking and forget the reasons we stopped. You may miss smoking, but don't kid yourself that smoking makes your life better. You know more effective ways to cope or celebrate, like taking a walk or talking to friends.

3. **Don't get cocky.** One of the worst things about cigarettes is their ability to snag their victims again. Don't give in to thoughts of *just one.*

4. **Be on the lookout and prepare for triggers.** By now you know which situations, people, and feelings are likely to tempt you to smoke. Keep using the skills that helped you cope in cutting down and quitting.

5. **Keep busy.** Many new ex-smokers have a hard time coping with boredom. Take up a new hobby, clean your closets, or paint the bathroom. Plan to

be busy. Don't sit around waiting for the smoking urge to grab you.

6. **Reward yourself.** Congratulations are in order each time you get through a milestone without smoking. After a week, give yourself a pat on the back and a reward. No matter how you do it, have fun and be good to yourself in some way. It helps to remind yourself that what you are doing is working.

7. **Think positive.** If negative thoughts start to creep in, remind yourself again that you are a nonsmoker, that you do not want to smoke, and that you have good reasons for it. Putting yourself down won't help. Positive thinking will.

8. **Relax.** Use breathing exercises to reduce tension. Instead of having a cigarette, take a long, deep breath, count to 5, and release it. Repeat until you've calmed down.

9. **Rely on support.** If you're thinking about reaching for a cigarette, reach for help instead. Ask your informal support group to congratulate you as you check off another day, week, and month as a nonsmoker; turn to your formal support group; or call your American Cancer Society at **800-227-2345**. We're here to support you.

Keep Up Your Guard

People often slip up and smoke again when they're either under extreme stress or while they're having a great time. If they're upset, they may think, "I used to smoke when I felt bad. Maybe a cigarette would make me feel better."

Or if they're happy, they may think, "I used to smoke when I was having fun. I bet a cigarette would help me have even more fun. I've been doing so well. I can go back to not smoking again tomorrow. Just one cigarette, just tonight."

If you find yourself rationalizing having a cigarette, stop! Remember, you're a nonsmoker now. That means not one puff! Nicotine is so addictive that it's impossible for most people to be occasional smokers. If you take even one puff off a cigarette, you're likely to start smoking again. The only way to be safe is not to smoke at all.

"When Have I Quit Forever?" The longer you've been a nonsmoker, the better your chances of remaining one. People who haven't smoked for a year have an 85 percent chance of remaining nonsmokers. Those who haven't smoked for 5 years have a 97 percent chance of staying off cigarettes. But there's never a guarantee that you've quit smoking forever. That's why keeping up your guard is important. People can quit for years, then smoke one cigarette and find themselves smoking regularly again.

When You're Tempted to Smoke

Even though you've made a commitment not to smoke, you'll sometimes be tempted to light up. Being a nonsmoker simply means not letting your cravings for a cigarette cause you to smoke.

Keep your list of reasons to quit in your wallet so you'll always have a copy when you feel the urge to smoke. Promise yourself that before you have a cigarette, you'll read through and consider each of the reasons you started to quit in the first place. Take a break and think for a few moments about all the hard work you've put into staying away from cigarettes.

Learn from Cravings. Instead of acting on your urges to smoke, keep learning from them. After you quit smoking, the urge to smoke often hits at predictable times. The trick is to anticipate those times and find ways to cope with them—without smoking. Think ahead to those times when you may be tempted to smoke, and plan on how you will use alternatives and activities to cope with these situations.

But remember, even if you slip, it doesn't mean an end to the nonsmoking you. It just means that you should figure out what triggered your slip, strengthen your commitment to quitting, and try again.

You've thought a lot about your triggers while reading this book. Don't forget about them now. Review the following sections:

- The "Why Test," pages 23–27
- "Break the Link," page 71
- "If You Used to Smoke When . . . ," pages 82–84

Regularly remind yourself of your personal triggers and how you plan to cope when you encounter them.

Be Prepared. You can expect and plan for many urges to smoke. But months or even years after you quit, you may feel an unexpected desire to smoke. To get through urges without smoking, try the following suggestions:

- Review your reasons for quitting and think of all the benefits to your health, your finances, and your family.

- Remind yourself that *there is no such thing as smoking just one cigarette*—or even one puff.

- Ride out the desire to smoke. It will go away whether you smoke or not.

▶ FACE TEMPTATION

For a few months after quitting, not smoking will take some getting use to. If you're ready for situations in which you could find yourself being pulled back to tobacco, you'll do fine.

Risky Situations

Times of Crisis

Troubles — like money problems, losing your job, or illness in the family — can bring on a strong urge to smoke.

Times of Celebration

Good times can trip you up just as bad ones can. You may be used to smoking at parties or as a treat when things are going well.

Down Times

You may have relied on cigarettes as your companion when you were lonely, depressed, or bored.

Time with Smokers

It's hard not to smoke when cigarettes are around, and it's even harder not to smoke when others are smoking. Some smokers may try to get you to have "just one."

Think of others times in your life when the urge to smoke will be strong and write them down. Make a plan for each of them. What will you do? What will you say?

(continued)

Ways to Handle It Without Tobacco

- Say to yourself, "A cigarette won't make this problem go away."

- Take a walk to give yourself a break and some time to think.

- Talk to someone about what you are going through.

- Pass up alcohol for a while. Dance, talk, and drink soda or juice.

- Don't give in to these smokers' thoughts:
  "I deserve a treat."
  "I'll just smoke 1 or 2 tonight."

- Remind yourself everyone has these moments.

- Do something active like clean out a closet, take a walk, or ride your bike.

- Get back into an old hobby or take up a new one.

- Pick up the phone and call an old friend.

- Spend less time with people who smoke.

- Stay away from smoky environments, like bars.

- Practice saying, "Thanks, I don't smoke."

Handle Stressful Situations. You've quit smoking, and you may be doing fine until—bam!—something stressful happens and you feel as though you have to have a cigarette to calm yourself down.

The steady stream of stress that flows day after day—things like missing the bus, arguing with the kids, facing a deadline at work, or having no milk for coffee—can be the greatest threat to living tobacco-free.

You've already learned many ways to manage stress without smoking. Find those that work for you, and make these methods of coping your new habits rather than falling back on cigarettes. Review the "Get a Handle

▶ WAYS TO HANDLE THE STRESS

These ideas may calm you down, give you a fresh outlook, and help you stay away from tobacco:

- **Have some fun.** Each day, find something you enjoy doing and make time for it. Build in "downtime" for relaxing.

- **Spend time with your support group.** Gravitate toward people who care about you in your new life as a nonsmoker.

- **Take care of yourself.** Try to eat well and get enough sleep. Keeping your body strong makes it easier to handle stress.

- **Get moving.** Research proves that regular exercise improves your mood and calms you down.

- **Try deep breathing.** It's simple, but it works if you need help in a hurry. When you are under stress, you often start to take shallow, rapid breaths without even knowing it.

on Stress" section on pages 66–67 to remind yourself of specific coping methods.

Celebrate without Smoking. Many people's smoking urges are linked to eating, celebrating, and drinking. And most people's urges occur when they're around other smokers. Stick to these tips for preventing urges:

- **Eat well without overindulging.** Pigging out can spark a tendency to overindulge on a regular basis.

- **Stretch out meals.** Eating slowly and pausing between bites will make the meal more satisfying.

- **Keep busy.** Play host or hostess, serve snacks, and greet guests to keep your mind off smoking.

- **Stay away from alcohol.** If you do drink alcohol, always choose a nonalcoholic drink first. Then water down your alcoholic drinks and put plenty of ice in them.

Spend Time with Nonsmoking Friends. When you first quit, it can be too much temptation to spend time with smoking friends. If coffee breaks at work were really smoke breaks, avoid the usual group for a while. If you rejoin them, expect to feel cravings and expect to be offered tobacco. If you can, create nonsmoking times to spend with friends who smoke.

Chart Your Progress

Think back over your quit attempt so far. Are you having as many withdrawal pangs or cravings as you did at first? How much time do you spend thinking about tobacco now? If you're having cravings for 10 minutes or so every couple of hours, think about this: You're doing just fine for 110 minutes of those 120.

Reward Yourself for Reaching Milestones

Reminding yourself of all the milestones you've reached can help inspire you to continue fighting off the smoking habit. Celebrate your first smoke-free week, your first smoke-free month, your first smoke-free birthday, and any other milestone you can think of.

In "Plan Rewards for Yourself," page 73, and "Treat Yourself," page 94, you thought of small ways to reward yourself for not smoking each day. As you look to the rest of your life, can you think of big ways to reward yourself for stopping smoking? What about redecorating and getting rid of smoke-stained wallpaper and rugs that never lose the smell of stale smoke? Or going on a weekend hiking trip and enjoying your ability to breathe and move more easily?

Daily Rewards *How can I reward myself each day for not smoking?*	Big Rewards *How can I reward myself after each smoke-free milestone?*
	One month:
	Three months:
	Six months:
	One year:

▶ IF YOU SMOKE AGAIN

If you do smoke a cigarette, don't be discouraged. Almost everyone who has tried to stop smoking has faced this moment of truth. Many give up and go back to smoking regularly, but you don't have to join them. Keep slip-ups in perspective and learn from them.

Rather than using a slip as an excuse to go back to smoking, look at what went wrong and renew your commitment to staying off smoking for good. The difference between a slip (a one-time loss of control) and a relapse (a return to regular smoking) is within your control.

- **A small setback doesn't mean you've become a smoker again.** Your very first cigarette didn't make you a smoker, and a small setback doesn't mean you are a smoker again.

- **Don't buy a pack because you have smoked 1 or 2 cigarettes.** Remember that you got through several days, or maybe even weeks or months, without a cigarette. This shows that you don't need cigarettes and that you can be a successful quitter.

- **Don't be too hard on yourself.** One slip doesn't mean you are a failure or that you can't be a nonsmoker. Tell yourself, "I'm not going to let all of this effort go to waste. I am still a nonsmoker!"

- **Learn from the experience.** What caused you to smoke? Boredom? Stress? How will you cope with a similar situation in the future?

(continued)

- **Know and use the coping skills in this book.**
  People who know at least one coping skill are more likely to remain nonsmokers than those who do not know any.

- **If you think you need professional help with quitting, see your doctor.** He or she can provide extra motivation for you to stop smoking. Your doctor may also prescribe a form of nicotine replacement or other medicine that helps you break your pattern of smoking.

If you've begun smoking again, don't give up! Many smokers can expect setbacks or relapses; it's a normal part of quitting. Some smokers try to quit multiple times before they quit for good. But studies show that each time you try to quit, you're more likely to succeed.

Review past attempts and identify what worked and what didn't so you can use your most successful strategies again. Any attempt to quit is a step in a healthier direction. When you feel ready to commit to quit again, review "My Most Recent Quit Attempt," pages 17–19, set a new Quit Day, and resolve to make your next attempt your last. No ifs, ands, or butts.

Stay Focused on Your Goals

Stopping smoking may be the hardest thing you've ever done, but you're well on your way to staying quit for good.

You've read this book, and you can always come back to it for tips on staying smoke-free for life. Don't leave all of this behind and go it alone. You're getting stronger every day, but everyone who quits can use reminders and refreshers in how to stay motivated. Some important sections to review regularly are listed here: "My Quitting Reminders," pages 20–21, "If You Used to Smoke When . . . ," pages 82–84, and "Daily Checklist," pages 92–93.

You've worked hard to become a nonsmoker. Since you quit, your life expectancy has increased, the food you eat tastes better, your clothes smell better, you've saved money, and you can breathe easier.

Now that you've set yourself free from cigarettes, celebrate all of the time and energy you've invested in the new you. Sit back and catch your breath. You're on the road to a healthier, happier life. You did it!

A Helping Hand

How to Support a Loved One Who's Quitting Smoking

SIGNIFICANT OTHERS AND FRIENDS don't always know how they can help a loved one quit smoking. This set of guidelines can help people support someone they care about during a quit attempt. Feel free to copy this list and keep it handy so you can help your loved one.

- Understand that this may be the toughest thing your loved one has ever done.

- Suggest nonsmoking activities you and your loved one can do together.

- Be patient if your loved one is irritable, distracted, or a little down when he or she quits. Smokers may go through withdrawal from the drug nicotine, but withdrawal symptoms are temporary.

- Ask your loved one to rely on you for support if he or she feels the urge to smoke. Make a deal with your loved one that he or she will call you before lighting up.

- Be a walking, running, or exercise class buddy.

- Remind your loved one regularly that you're proud of him or her.

- Celebrate your loved one's nonsmoking milestones with him or her. Ask what you can do to reward your loved one's achievements.

- Remind your loved one of all the benefits to his or her health, wallet, and self-image.

- If you're a smoker, don't smoke around your loved one. Keep cigarettes out of sight and out of reach when your loved one is around.

- Ask your loved one about his or her biggest challenges to staying smoke free—whether during coffee breaks, after lunch, at the end of the workday, or when feeling stress, for example—and offer to check in at those times.

- Be a custom-made support person . . . ask exactly how you can help keep your loved one on a nonsmoking track.

- Don't nag or make your loved one feel guilty if he or she slips up or struggles with quitting. Support your loved one through challenges or as he or she tries again.

Resource Guide

A VARIETY OF ORGANIZATIONS offer information on how to quit and where to go for help. If you want to quit smoking and you need help, talk with your health care provider and contact one of the organizations here. Together they can provide you with current information, advice, and suggestions for ending your tobacco use. You may also want to call your state's Department of Health to see if they offer a state-sponsored stop-smoking program.

American Cancer Society Resources

American Cancer Society
Toll-Free: **800-227-2345** Web site: **cancer.org**
The American Cancer Society is the nationwide community-based volunteer health organization dedicated to eliminating cancer as a major health problem by preventing cancer, saving lives, and diminishing suffering from cancer through research, education, advocacy, and service. Call **800-227-2345** or visit **cancer.org** to locate your division office for your state or region, or for more information about smoking cessation or cancer-related topics. The publications listed in the back of this book are available for sale through the Society's toll-free number and Web site and include information about general health, cancer, and prevention.

Self-Help Materials
Materials are available to help you quit smoking, no matter where you are in the process. You can use the materials to learn how to prepare for your quit attempt, develop

strategies to help with cravings, and prevent relapsing once you have quit. Self-help materials offer proven methods that are easy to follow and can keep your motivation high. The American Cancer Society's "Break Away from the Pack" series has been shown to double your chances of quitting successfully. For more information on "Break Away from the Pack" or other self-help materials from the American Cancer Society, call **800-227-2345**.

Community Resources

The American Cancer Society can tell you about smoking cessation resources in your community. These may include classes, support groups, Internet resources, or medication assistance referrals. It is important to have support from several different sources during your quit attempt, including family, friends, doctors, and cessation professionals. Call **800-227-2345** for more details.

Quitlines (Telephone Counseling Programs)

You may be able to use a telephone counseling program, or quitline, in your area. You can receive quitting strategies and support over the phone, at times that are convenient for you. Quitlines have been proven to double your chances of successfully quitting. Your state may sponsor a quitline, or you can call the American Cancer Society at **800-227-2345** for information about smoking cessation programs.

The Great American Smokeout

The American Cancer Society's Great American Smokeout is a special day set aside to motivate smokers to quit for a day—and hopefully stay off cigarettes for a lifetime. Through the Great American Smokeout and other year-round tobacco cessation programs and services, the Society continues to inform people about the dangers of smoking and tobacco use and to save lives by providing the tools to help users quit. For more information about how to get involved in the Great American Smokeout and to learn about tobacco cessation strategies, visit us at **cancer.org**.

Other Organizations and Resources

The American Cancer Society does not necessarily endorse the agencies, organizations, corporations, and publications represented in this resource guide. This guide is provided for assistance in obtaining information only.

American Lung Association (ALA)

61 Broadway, 6th Floor
New York, NY 10006
Toll-free: 800-548-8252
Telephone: 212-315-8700
Fax: 212-265-5642
Web site: *http://www.lungusa.org*

ALA is a voluntary, nonprofit agency fighting lung diseases. Its mission is to prevent lung disease and promote lung health, with special emphasis on asthma, tobacco control, and environmental health. The ALA Web site provides detailed information about lung diseases, information about ALA programs and events, a list of publications, and an ALA chapter locator.

Foundation for a Smokefree America

P. O. Box 492028
Los Angeles, CA 90049-8028
Telephone: 310-471-0303
Web site: *http://www.anti-smoking.org*

Created by Patrick Reynolds (grandson of R. J. Reynolds), the Foundation for a Smokefree America is a nonprofit group whose mission is to educate people of all ages about smoking and tobacco use. The Web sites *AntiSmoking.org*, *NoTobacco.org*, and *TobaccoFree.org* have information about smoking and quitting tips.

Nicotine Anonymous World Services

419 Main Street, PMB #370
Huntington Beach, CA 92648
Telephone: 415-750-0328
Web site: *http://www.nicotine-anonymous.org*

Nicotine Anonymous is an anonymous support group, based on a twelve-step fellowship, of people who want to live free of nicotine addiction. The Web site provides nicotine cessation and support literature in five languages, answers to frequently asked questions about nicotine addiction, and a worldwide list of meetings.

The Office on Smoking and Health (OSH)

National Center for Chronic Disease Prevention and Health Promotion/CDC
4770 Buford Highway NE, Mail Stop K-40
Atlanta, GA 30341-3717
Toll-Free: 800-CDC-1311 (800-232-4636)
Web site: *http://www.cdc.gov/tobacco*

This Centers for Disease Control and Prevention office is a division within the National Center for Chronic Disease Prevention and Health Promotion within the U.S. Department of Health and Human Services. OSH is responsible for leading and coordinating strategic efforts aimed at preventing tobacco use among youth, promoting tobacco cessation, and protecting nonsmokers from environmental tobacco smoke (ETS). The Web site offers public education and information on smoking and how to stop.

QuitNet

1 Appleton Street, 4th floor
Boston, MA 02116
Telephone: 617-437-1500
Fax: 617-437-9394
Web site: *http://www.quitnet.org*

QuitNet.com, Inc. is a private company operating in association with Boston University School of Public Health. It provides cutting edge, effective tobacco cessation services to people worldwide. The Web site includes chat rooms, quitting guides, quitting calendars, a national directory of local smoking cessation programs, tobacco news, and personalized services like peer-to-peer support, tools to track your progress and recommend strategies, and access to online counselors. Registration is required, and some services require a fee.

The Robert Wood Johnson Foundation (RWJF)
P. O. Box 2316
Route 1 College Road
East Princeton, NJ 08543-2316
Toll-Free: 877-843-7953
Web site: *http://www.rwjf.org*

RWJF was established as a national philanthropy and is the largest U.S. foundation devoted to improving the health and health care of all Americans. In 1994, it created the program Smoke-Free Families (SFF): Innovations to Stop Smoking During and Beyond Pregnancy (*http://www.smokefree families.org*).

World No Tobacco Day (WNTD)
World Health Organization
Regional Office for the Americas/Pan American Health Organization
525 23rd Street NW
Washington, DC 20037
Telephone: 202-974-3000 (Main)
Telephone: 202-974-3457 (Office of Public Information)
Telephone: 212-601-8245 for information about
World No Tobacco Day
Fax: 202-974-3663
Web site: *http://www.wntd.com*

The World Health Organization annually sponsors WNTD to call attention to the seriousness of the impact of tobacco on health. WNTD is the first and only global event where smokers around the world unite to break free from their dependence on tobacco. First held in 1988, and observed annually on May 31, WNTD is the only global event established to raise awareness of the international impact of tobacco use and promote a tobacco-free environment.

Glossary

acetylcholine (ah-SEH-tel-co-leen): a signal transmitter in the nervous system.

acupuncture: a Chinese medical practice in which needles are inserted at specified sites in the body to treat illness or provide local anesthesia. Acupuncture for smoking is usually done on certain parts of the ears. Despite the suggestion that acupuncture can lower the desire to smoke, there is no solid evidence that it is effective for smoking cessation.

addiction: the condition of being compulsively occupied with or involved in a habit-forming substance, characterized by tolerance and by well-defined physiological symptoms upon withdrawal. *See also* withdrawal.

atropine (AH-tro-peen) and scopolamine (SKO-pol-a-meen) combination therapy: a smoking cessation therapy used by some clinics to reduce nicotine withdrawal symptoms. Therapy involves injections of atropine and scopolamine. These drugs block the action of acetylcholine, a signal transmitter in the nervous system.

Note: Both atropine and scopolamine are FDA-approved for other uses, but have not been approved for help in quitting smoking.

bupropion (bu-PRO-pee-on): a non-nicotine, prescription drug originally used to treat depression, now commonly used as a stop-smoking aid that helps reduce nicotine cravings. The brand name is Zyban.

carbon monoxide (CO): a compound made up of molecules containing one carbon atom and one oxygen atom, which produces a colorless, odorless, poisonous gas, often when a material burns. Cigarette smoke can contain high levels of carbon monoxide.

clonidine (KLON-a-deen): an older medicine used to treat high blood pressure. When used for smoking cessation, it can be taken in the form of a pill, twice a day, or as a skin patch, applied once a week. Clonidine has been recommended by the Agency for Healthcare Research and Quality (AHRQ) for smoking cessation, but it has not been approved by the FDA for this purpose.

cold turkey: to abruptly stop use of an addictive substance.

cotinine (CO-teh-neen): a compound that results when nicotine is broken down in the body; a "by-product" of nicotine, widely used as an indicator of recent exposure to the substance.

cravings: a consuming desire or yearning for nicotine as a result of withdrawal. *See also* withdrawal.

dietary supplement: a product (other than tobacco) that is intended to supplement the diet and contains one or more of the following ingredients: a vitamin, a mineral, an herb or other botanical, an amino acid.

electronic cigarette: a refillable cartridge designed to look like a cigarette, which delivers a mist of liquid, flavorings, and nicotine resembling smoke. Nicotine is absorbed into the lungs when the smoker inhales this mist. The electronic cigarette is not an FDA-approved method of nicotine replacement.

FDA: *See* U.S. Food and Drug Administration.

habit: an acquired, often unconscious pattern of behavior regularly followed until it has become almost involuntary.

hypnosis (hip-NOH-sis): an altered state of consciousness that is artificially induced and characterized by increased susceptibility to suggestion. Studies of hypnosis to help people quit smoking have not produced sufficient evidence that this is a reliable quitting method.

low-level laser therapy: an acupuncture technique in which cold lasers are used instead of needles to stimulate the body's acupoints. The treatment is supposed to relax the smoker and release pain relief substances in the body that mimic the effects of nicotine in the brain or balance the body's energy to relieve the addiction. *See also* acupuncture.

nicotine (NICK-o-teen): a colorless, poisonous compound occurring naturally in the tobacco plant. It is the substance in tobacco to which smokers can become addicted. *See also* addiction.

nicotine gum: a fast-acting method of nicotine replacement therapy that is available without a prescription. Chewing the gum releases nicotine, which is then absorbed through the lining of the mouth. Also called nicotine polacrilex.

nicotine inhaler: a method of nicotine replacement that uses a plastic tube about the size of a cigarette with a nicotine cartridge inside. When placed in the mouth, the cartridge delivers nicotine through an inhaled vapor. One inhaler cartridge contains about the same amount of nicotine found in two cigarettes. Nicotine inhalers are available by prescription only.

nicotine lip balm: *See* nicotine salicylate.

nicotine lollipops: *See* nicotine salicylate.

nicotine lozenges: small capsules or tablets available as an over-the-counter form of nicotine replacement therapy. The lozenge releases nicotine as it slowly dissolves. The nicotine is absorbed into the bloodstream through the lining of the mouth.

nicotine nasal spray: an aerosol spray form of nicotine replacement. When sprayed into the nostrils, this method quickly sends nicotine to the bloodstream. Nicotine nasal spray is available by prescription only.

nicotine patch: a method of nicotine replacement in which an adhesive patch is stuck to the skin to provide a constant, measured dose of nicotine. The nicotine enters the blood through the skin and reaches the bloodstream over several hours. Nicotine will continue to enter the bloodstream several hours after the patch is removed. The patch is available over the counter, without a prescription. Also called a nicotine transdermal system.

nicotine polacrilex: *See* nicotine gum.

nicotine replacement therapy: various tobacco cessation methods designed to take the place of cigarettes, cigars, snuff, and pipes in delivering nicotine to the body, These products come in the form of gum, lozenges, nasal sprays, inhalers, and patches. *See also* nicotine gum, nicotine lozenges, nicotine nasal spray, nicotine patch.

nicotine salicylate (NICK-o-teen sa-LISS-uh-late): a form of nicotine replacement that is available in both a lollipop and a lip balm. These products have not been approved by the FDA for use in smoking cessation, and sales of these products are prohibited in the United States.

nicotine transdermal systems: *See* nicotine patch.

nicotine wafer: a thin disk made of a food-grade edible paper infused with nicotine. When the wafer is placed in the mouth, nicotine is absorbed rapidly through the tissues under the tongue or behind the lower lip. This product is advertised as a way to get a nicotine "fix" in places where smoking is not allowed, but it is not an aid to smoking cessation.

nicotine water: bottled water with added nicotine to match the amount contained in two to three cigarettes. This product is advertised as a way to get a nicotine "fix" in places where smoking is not allowed and is not considered a smoking cessation aid.

nortriptyline (nor-TRIP-tah-leen): an older antidepressant prescription medicine recommended by the

Agency for Healthcare Research and Quality (AHRQ) to help people quit smoking. Nortriptyline has not been approved by the FDA for this "off-label" purpose.

snuff: a preparation of tobacco, either powdered and taken into the nostrils by inhalation or chewed and placed between the cheek and gums.

tobacco (tah-BACK-oh): a plant with leaves that have high levels of the addictive chemical nicotine. The leaves may be smoked (in cigarettes, cigars, and pipes), applied to the gums (as dipping and chewing tobacco), or inhaled (as snuff). Tobacco leaves also contain many cancer-causing chemicals, and tobacco use and exposure to secondhand tobacco smoke have been linked to many types of cancer and other diseases. The scientific name is *Nicotiana tabacum*.

tobacco lozenges: small capsules or tablets, often flavored, that contain tobacco. Sold as an alternative to smoking for users to get nicotine in places where smoking is not allowed. Tobacco lozenges are not considered smoking cessation aids. Brand names include Ariva and Interval.

tobacco pouches: miniature tea-bag–like pockets containing tobacco sold as an alternative to smoking for users to get nicotine in places where smoking is not allowed. The user places the pouch between the cheek and the gums, and nicotine is absorbed through the lining of the mouth. Tobacco pouches are not considered smoking cessation aids. Brand names include Revel and Exalt.

tolerance: the lessening of the physiological response to a substance that occurs after continued use, requiring larger doses to produce a given response.

trigger: an action or experience that stimulates the desire to smoke.

varenicline (ver-EN-eh-kleen): a newer prescription medicine for smoking cessation, which is taken in pill form. Varenicline interferes with nicotine receptors in the brain. It lessens the pleasurable physical effects of smoking and reduces symptoms of nicotine withdrawal. The brand name is Chantix.

U.S. Food and Drug Administration (FDA): an agency of the United States Department of Health and Human Services. The FDA is responsible for regulating tobacco, drugs, biological medical products, blood products, medical devices, and radiation-emitting devices, along with several other categories of products.

withdrawal: stopping the use of an addictive substance; often accompanied by physiological and psychological effects brought on by the absence of that substance.

Index

Books Published by the American Cancer Society

Available everywhere books are sold and online at **cancer.org/bookstore**

Information

The American Cancer Society: A History of Saving Lives

American Cancer Society's Complete Guide to Colorectal Cancer

American Cancer Society Complete Guide to Complementary & Alternative Cancer Therapies, Second Edition

American Cancer Society Complete Guide to Nutrition for Cancer Survivors: Eating Well, Staying Well During and After Cancer, Second Edition

Breast Cancer Clear & Simple: All Your Questions Answered

The Cancer Atlas (available in English, Spanish, French, and Chinese)

Cancer: What Causes It, What Doesn't

QuickFACTS™—Advanced Cancer

QuickFACTS™—Bone Metastasis

QuickFACTS™—Colorectal Cancer, Second Edition

QuickFACTS™—Lung Cancer

QuickFACTS™—Prostate Cancer, Second Edition

QuickFACTS™—Thyroid Cancer

The Tobacco Atlas, Third Edition (available in English, Spanish, French, and Chinese)

Day-to-Day Help

American Cancer Society's Guide to Pain Control: Understanding and Managing Cancer Pain, Revised Edition

Cancer Caregiving A to Z: An At-Home Guide for Patients and Families

Caregiving: A Step-By-Step Resource for Caring for the Person with Cancer at Home, Revised Edition

Get Better! Communication Cards for Kids & Adults

Lymphedema: Understanding and Managing Lymphedema After Cancer Treatment

Social Work in Oncology: Supporting Survivors, Families and Caregivers

What to Eat During Cancer Treatment: 100 Great-Tasting, Family-Friendly Recipes to Help You Cope

When the Focus Is on Care: Palliative Care and Cancer

Emotional Support

Angels & Monsters: A child's eye view of cancer

Cancer in the Family: Helping Children Cope with a Parent's Illness

Chemo and Me: My Hair Loss Experience

Couples Confronting Cancer: Keeping Your Relationship Strong

Crossing Divides: A Couple's Story of Cancer, Hope, and Hiking Montana's Continental Divide

I Can Survive

The Survivorship Net: A Parable for the Family, Friends, and Caregivers of People with Cancer

What Helped Get Me Through: Cancer Survivors Share Wisdom and Hope

Just for Kids

Because . . . Someone I Love Has Cancer: Kids' Activity Book

Healthy Me: A Read-Along Coloring & Activity Book

Jacob Has Cancer: His Friends Want to Help

Kids' First Cookbook: Delicious-Nutritious Treats To Make Yourself!

Let My Colors Out

Mom and the Polka-Dot Boo-Boo

Nana, What's Cancer?

No Thanks, but I'd Love to Dance

Our Dad Is Getting Better

Our Mom Has Cancer (hardcover)

Our Mom Has Cancer (paperback)

Our Mom Is Getting Better

What's Up with Bridget's Mom? Medikidz Explain Breast Cancer

What's Up with Richard? Medikidz Explain Leukemia

Prevention

The American Cancer Society's Healthy Eating Cookbook: A Celebration of Food, Friendship, and Healthy Living, Third Edition

Celebrate! Healthy Entertaining for Any Occasion

Good for You! Reducing Your Risk of Developing Cancer

The Great American Eat-Right Cookbook: 140 Great-Tasting, Good-for-You Recipes

Healthy Air: A Read-Along Coloring & Activity Book (25 per pack: Tobacco avoidance)

Healthy Bodies: A Read-Along Coloring & Activity Book (25 per pack: Physical activity)

Healthy Food: A Read-Along Coloring & Activity Book (25 per pack: Nutrition)

National Health Education Standards: Achieving Excellence, Second Edition (available in paperback and on CD-ROM)

Reduce Your Cancer Risk: Twelve Steps to a Healthier Life